Lose Weight
for
LIFE
LISA RILEY

MICHAEL JOSEPH
an imprint of
PENGUIN BOOKS

To Al. *We always say 'if you know, you know'. The best thing is: we do know! You never cease to amaze me when it comes to pure, honest support. Forever blessed, forever grateful, forever loved. That's the best journey.*

To my family. *For always being the butt of every good joke. I simply say the family that plays together stays together. Let the laughter (and the carbs!) live on.*

To my beloved angel. *I never tire of writing this. I know you are with me and would be so eternally proud. That keeps my smile as wide as it can be, just like yours. I love you, Mum, every second of every single day.*

MICHAEL JOSEPH
UK | USA | Canada | Ireland | Australia
India | New Zealand | South Africa

Michael Joseph is part of the Penguin Random House group of companies whose addresses can be found at global.penguinrandomhouse.com

Penguin
Random House
UK

First published 2018
001

Text copyright © Lisa Riley, 2018
Food photography © Clare Winfield, 2018

The moral right of the copyright holders has been asserted

Edited by Jordan Paramor
Design and layout by HART STUDIO
Hair and make-up by Tracey Jones and Bekki Mitchell
Food styling and recipe development by Kat Mead
Prop styling by Jemima Hetherington

Colour reproduction by Altaimage Ltd
Printed in Germany by Mohn Media

A CIP catalogue record for this book is available from the British Library

ISBN: 978–0–241–34912–0

www.greenpenguin.co.uk

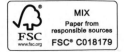

Penguin Random House is committed to a sustainable future for our business, our readers and our planet. This book is made from Forest Stewardship Council® certified paper.

Photography of author © Nicky Johnston, except p38 (right) © Ken McKay/REX/Shutterstock; (bottom) © David M. Benett/Getty Images

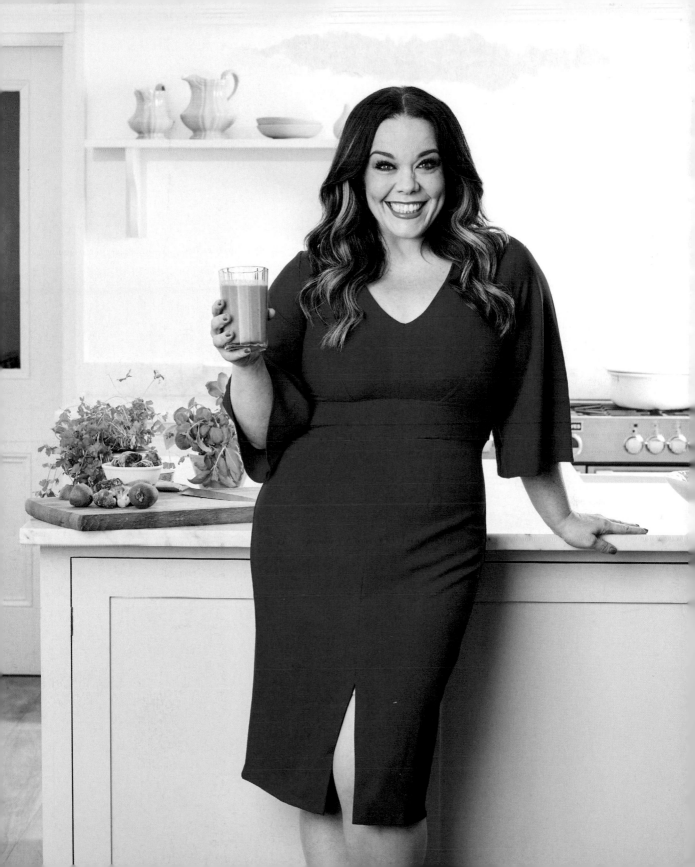

Lose Weight
for
LIFE

CONTENTS

THE DIET PLAN

THE RECIPES

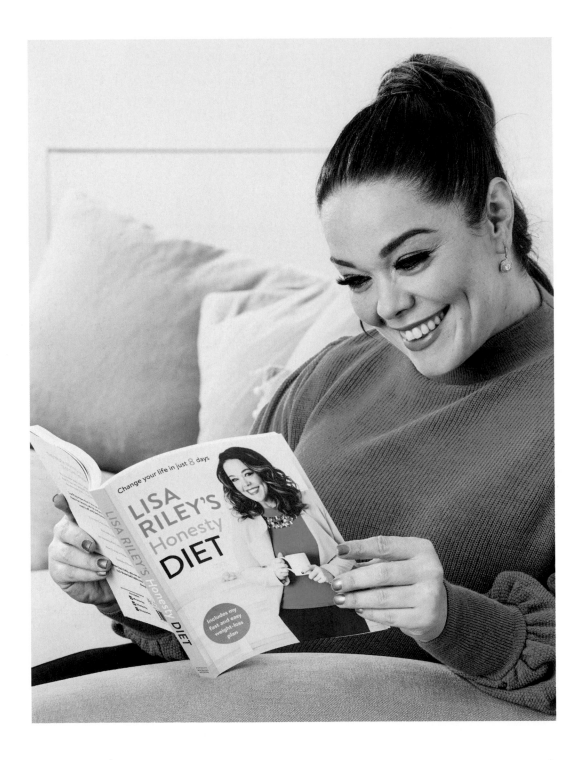

INTRODUCTION

Hi, everyone! It's great to have you here. If you're new to my books, I really hope you're about to find the inspiration and motivation you're searching for. If you've read my *Honesty Diet* and you're back for more, I'm impressed! I hope you'll love this book every bit as much as you did the first.

I've stepped things up a bit in Book Two, and as well as bringing you loads of lovely new recipes and kick-ass workout plans to help keep things fun, interesting and easy to stick to, it's all about taking you to the next stage of healthy living, re-emphasizing the importance of honesty, and learning how to take care of yourself in the way that you should:

- emotionally
- physically
- for the long term

Losing weight begins as much in your head and heart as it does in the gym or the kitchen. You have to like and respect yourself enough to know that you're worthy of feeling amazing every single day of your life. In the pages of this book you'll find tons of tools that will help you to do exactly that.

This isn't a fast fix, this is about forever.

As you may already know, my body transformation has been achieved by eating good foods, smaller portions and working out regularly. But if I hadn't got my head into the right space to begin with, none of that would or could have happened. If you've already had success with tackling your thinking using my Honesty Diet and you feel like you're ready to take things to the next level, or if you're worrying you've backtracked or plateaued a bit lately, in this book you will find loads of helpful mental strategies to help you to up your game.

Since losing weight I've worked just as much on keeping a positive mindset as I have on making healthy choices and ensuring my bum stays firm. I do that by constantly reminding myself of how I got from where I was to where I am now, and by actively learning new ways to keep myself on track. Whether it's by writing a gratitude list or reading positive affirmations on social media (I also keep an extensive collection on my phone!), training my brain to think positive is a daily priority for me. I want to show you how to do the same.

You are going to love this book if:

- You've been dieting on and off for many years and don't believe you'll ever truly be able to lose weight. You can – and I'm going to show you how making just a few simple changes can help you keep the weight off for life.

- You think your body has been ruined by years of yo-yo dieting and can never look good again. It can and it will. Just look at me!

- You're confused by all the mixed dieting and exercise messages that are out there. Forget all that! I like to keep things simple and keep them real.

- You kick-started your healthy lifestyle journey with my Honesty Diet and now you want to step things up, try some delicious new recipes and discover brilliant new techniques to store in your weight-loss locker.

You are going to do this, because you're amazing and you deserve to.

Believe me when I say that anything is possible. Three years ago I was twelve stone heavier than I am now. That's a whole person. Now? I'm healthy, happy and embracing life to the fullest. Am I perfect? Absolutely not. Will I ever be? No, because there's no such thing. But I'm perfectly me, and every day I work on being the best I can be. And if I can do it, you can too.

Even supermodels and stunning celebrities have insecurities. You may think, 'Well, if they're not happy, what chance have I got?' But here's the thing – being happy with yourself is a choice.

Let today be the day when you choose to be kind to yourself and to your body.

If you've picked up this book, the chances are you think there's room for improvement and you'd like to lose weight and feel great. Or you might have read my first book, lost a bit of weight already (in which case, a huge Well Done!), but now your progress has slowed down and you're looking for more ideas and inspiration to help ramp things up again. Perhaps you found success with my first book and now you're looking for the next challenge. Brilliant, let's get to it!

Before we start, I want to say please, please, please don't give yourself a hard time at any point while you're reading my books or following my advice. Being negative will only hold you back. Instead of focusing on being unhappy with your body as it is right now, put all that energy into focusing on where you want to be, because that's where you're eventually going to be.

Why waste any more time wishing you were a certain size and feeling down because you're not? Let's just get on and do it! I'm going to teach you how to get your head into the best place, and before you know it your body will follow.

I'm so excited for you.

Lots of love, Lisa xxx

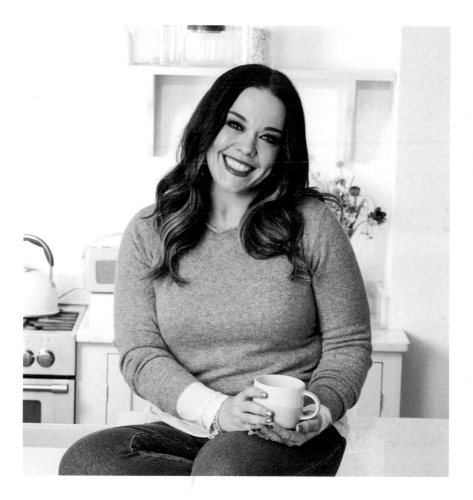

CHAPTER 1

Mind Matters

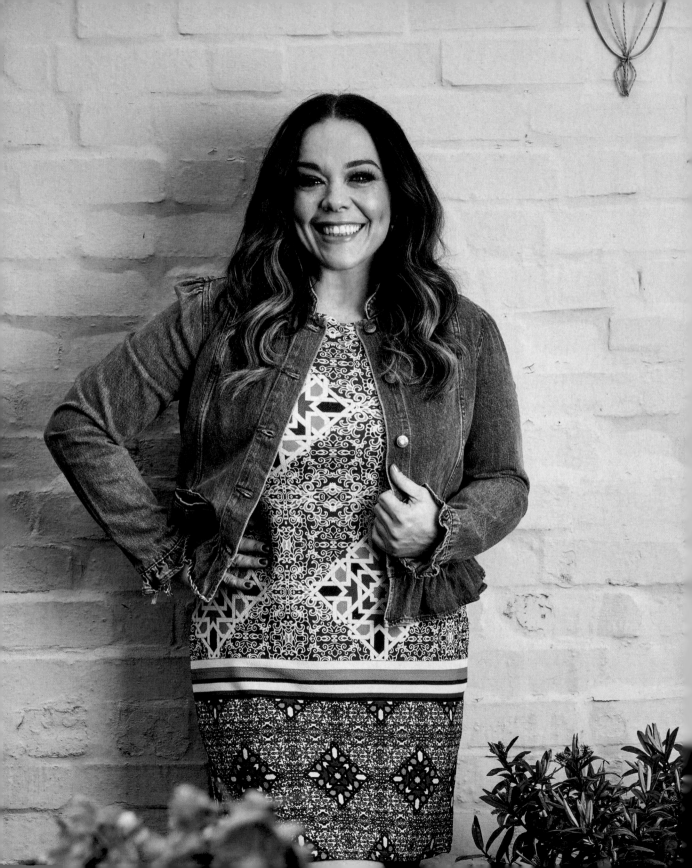

I want to kick off with this chapter because it's all about getting ourselves into a great place mentally, not to mention learning to love ourselves. And in my opinion they are two things which are essential when it comes to weight loss.

The irony for me is that the biggest struggle in keeping the weight off hasn't so much been physically, but that at times it's been a huge struggle mentally. In the early days, I often found it really hard to cope with how much I'd changed. Sometimes I still see myself as that other person – the old, overweight me. Even now I get days where I wonder if I'm doing enough, eating well enough, being a good enough person. But that's a part of being human, I guess. Then I'll have other days where I'll feel on top of the world and really positive and ready for whatever comes my way. It's about learning to go with how I'm feeling on a daily basis and giving myself a break if things go wrong or my workload means I don't manage as long in the gym as I'd wanted to.

My attitude used to be so bad at times that I would create problems for myself, and I would always imagine the worst-case scenarios, just in case they happened. For instance, I'd have arguments in my head with imaginary people who commented on my weight, even though no one ever did. I was so defensive. If I'm being honest, I think I felt a bit angry with the world. I thought it was unfair that I was so big, and that manifested itself as negativity. One recurring thought I had a lot was, 'If I lose weight, I'll only put it on again, so what's the point?' I was so sure it would all pile straight back on again that I didn't even give it a try. Imagine if I'd never challenged that thought? I would still be stuck in the same miserable place. I really do believe it was my decision to keep an Honesty Diary that helped me get past that blockage and find a way forward. I'm not saying it was an overnight thing, but by getting those thoughts and feelings down on paper I could start to make more sense of them.

There's an amazing saying that goes: 'Some people create their own storms and then complain when it rains.' I have to say, that was me at times. Once I was in a negative loop I didn't know how to get out of it again. It was only by finding a way to stop those thoughts, and dealing with my anger and resentment, that I was finally able to lose weight. You need to learn how to put the handbrake on negative thoughts. Only you are in control of that. Your partner, your husband, your wife, your kids, your best friend – they can all help – but not until you make the decision that you want to help yourself. No blame game please!

Only you can get yourself to the place you want to be, and only you can keep yourself there.

All the work I've done on myself mentally over the past couple of years has meant that I'm now so happy in myself that I love my own company, and that's something I wouldn't have been able to say a few years ago. If I spent time on my own in the old days, I would stew in my own negativity and quickly get into a really bad headspace. But now I know how to avoid that, whether by exercising, or writing in my journal, which as you know is so important to me. By writing things down you get them out, and that's why I'm going to be encouraging you to start or keep up with your Honesty Diary in the same way I did in my last book. It's an essential part of your weight loss, because it helps to challenge and change old patterns that no longer work for you. Believe me, if you don't do it, you will miss out on some important tools.

Here are some things you need to know about the journey we're about to start on.

WE'RE GOING TO LAYER ON THE GOODNESS!

Remember when you used to make a sandwich and layer it with butter and cheese and mayonnaise? Now you're going to layer goodness on yourself. You're going to tell yourself every day how much you deserve a happy, healthy, fulfilled life. In the same way you developed bad habits – such as overeating and not exercising – now you're going to teach yourself new ones, and it all starts with realizing just how bloody great you are. You are going to literally feed yourself love.

FIND WHAT DRIVES YOU

What drives me a lot is fear that I'll go back to my old ways – and I never want to go back there. It could be that you have a big event coming up, or that your health is suffering because of your weight and you're keen to improve it, or that you simply want to feel happier with how you look. Identify your motivations and write them down.

SELF-LOATHING WILL GET YOU NOWHERE

Self-hatred will not motivate you, and nor will it encourage your body to lose weight. If you try to bully yourself into change, you're coming at the whole process from a negative place. Rather than wasting energy trying not to hate yourself, learn to love yourself instead. If you walk past a news-stand and see a Hollywood actress looking incredible, don't think, 'I want to look like that and I won't be happy until I do.' You might as well hit yourself with a cricket bat. It's not realistic and it won't get you anywhere. Comparison-itis is so destructive. Besides, that celebrity probably exercises for five hours a day and has been heavily airbrushed. So take a tip from *Frozen's* Queen Elsa and 'Let it go.'

Every single person is unique, with no two fingerprints the same, and that's how you have to treat your body. It's so individual.

The wandering female eye in the gym changing room is legendary, and it's often when we suffer from comparison-itis the most. I genuinely don't look at other women when they're getting changed because I don't care what their bodies are like. I'm too busy telling myself how great mine is. Not perfect, but bloody great. You won't ever feel better about yourself by putting someone else down. If you do, it comes from a place of insecurity. Why should it make you feel better that someone else's bum is saggier than yours? Someone being bigger than you isn't going to make you thinner. It's going to make you feel toxic. I'm covered in scars, so what would they say about me!

Turn those thoughts around. Every time you find yourself being critical about someone, catch yourself and notice something positive about them instead. Maybe they've got nice hair? Maybe you like their sense of style? Trust me, it will make a big difference. If you can stop judging other people, you can stop judging yourself too. It really is crucial.

CRYING IS GOOD

Never feel bad about crying. Crying helps to get everything out and release all those emotions that you're holding on to and bottling up. It's obvious but so, so true. Never apologize for being upset. Crying is a detox in the same way that sneezing, coughing, blowing your nose and farting are. All of that stuff has got to come out. It's completely normal. If you're feeling weepy, don't hold it in – you'll probably end up going and grabbing a Twix to make yourself feel better.

I was on a plane flying via Canada a while back, and because I lived there as a child, all of a sudden this massive wave of emotion about my mum's death crashed over me. I burst out crying, to the point where I couldn't control it, and I was so worried about what the people sitting around me would think. Then I got over that and thought, 'This is the most natural thing in the world.' I was missing my mum and I needed to express how I was feeling.

If I hadn't let that pain out, it would have festered and I could easily have spent the nine hours on that plane chewing away not only at those thoughts but also at any food that came my way. Think about how bad it feels when you're desperate for the loo and there's nowhere to go. Treat tears the same way and release them. Even if you're crying about not being able to eat a giant bag of chocolate buttons, embrace those tears. If in doubt, put a weepy film on and have a bloody good sob.

DON'T PANIC ABOUT PANICKING

Some degree of panic or worry is normal. It's part of everyday life, and it's something that existed right back in caveman times when people were being chased by dinosaurs. I don't know about you, but I would feel pretty panicked if a bloody great Tyrannosaurus Rex was running after me because he wanted to make me his dinner!

I know from experience that anxiety can lead to snacking. I used to suffer horrendously from panic attacks when I was in *Emmerdale*. For a while, I lost track of whether I was Mandy Dingle or Lisa Riley. I'd film all day and then go and do an appearance in the evening and no one wanted to see me, they wanted to see my character. They wanted that loud tomboy character, so I'd 'turn on' Mandy when I was in front of the mike. When I wasn't at work I was often learning lines, and I went through a phase of spending more hours as Mandy than I did as Lisa, and ultimately not knowing who I really was. That took its toll on me and I ended up feeling very anxious. It was before I discovered the magic of keeping diaries, so everything used to go round and round in my head. I didn't have a way to release it, apart from by eating or drinking a lot of rubbish, which didn't help matters. Sugar can trigger a rise in your heart rate, which might make you feel more panicky. It may seem like a short-term fix but that bar of chocolate will only make things worse.

When the panic attacks hit, I used to feel like someone was pushing on my chest and I was going to have a heart attack. I would not wish panic attacks on my worst enemy. They are horrible things. I was on holiday once and had a massive panic attack. The resort had to call a doctor and I had an injection of Valium in my bottom. I was panicking about panicking, and I was so caught up in it I couldn't get myself out of it. It was Mother Nature telling me to calm down and train my thoughts.

I do have a busy brain generally, and I also have a fertile imagination where I create scenarios in my head – even when they're not there (see my comments about imaginary arguments earlier!) – and sometimes I invent situations that cause me anxiety. Whereas I used to grab a paper bag and breathe into it, or wolf down a giant pizza, now I write down how I'm feeling and by doing that I make sense of it. If I can, I'll also get myself out of the house and go for a walk. Or I'll do an exercise DVD or class to get it out of my system. I replace anxiety or upset with the high I get from exercising.

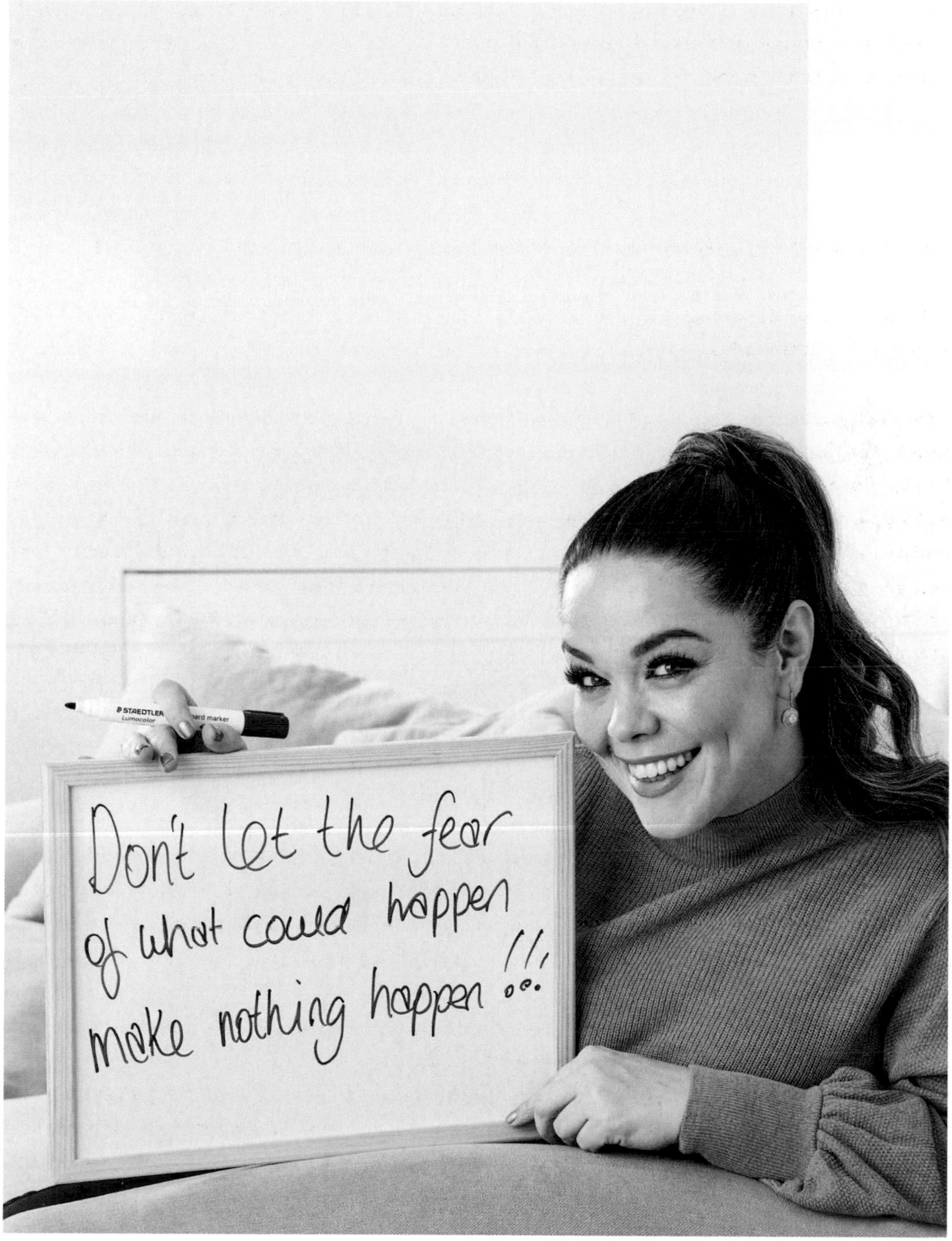
Don't let the fear
of what could happen
make nothing happen !!!

YOU ARE NEVER TOO OLD TO FEEL
GOOD ABOUT YOURSELF

In my opinion, life is getting better as I get older. There is no age limit to when you can look and feel good. Confidence is often the key to looking good, and that definitely comes with age and being comfortable in your skin. If you feel better about yourself at fifty than you did at twenty, it will show. You will glow. It doesn't matter if you have a bit more cellulite – or some smile lines (a much nicer term for wrinkles!) – you can still walk into a room and own it.

A good friend of mine is like a magnet to people. She's in her early forties and a curvy size 14. She has to go to a lot of functions for work and she said to me recently, 'When I walk into a room, I know I'm probably not going to be the youngest, the prettiest or the slimmest person in there, but I know I'm going to be one of the most confident, and as a result I'll be one of the most fun and most interesting. Because of that I spend the evening surrounded by people. In my twenties I felt like I had to compete with other women my age and I felt inferior if they were a size 10. Now? I don't compete with anyone, because I feel great about who I am.'

How amazing is that? I, too, find that I care much less about what people think these days. It's such a relief! You can't please everyone all the time, and I'm certainly not going to feel bad about myself because I'm over forty. There are so many incredible, sexy older women around. If you're in that age bracket, why not be one of them?

BE KIND TO YOUR BODY

Something my wound recovery (after my skin-removal surgery) did for me was help me to really get in touch with my body, more than I ever have. Just the ritual of putting arnica cream on my scars every day made me feel like I was taking great care of myself. I was literally loving my body as I was rubbing it in. I was helping my body to heal and feel better.

I suspect that 99 per cent of people who have had body or eating issues over the years have lost touch with their body. Instead of feeling grateful to it they feel angry with it, so they don't take care of it like they once did. If you feel like that, the first thing I would recommend is to start properly pampering yourself. I don't mean going off to posh overpriced spas or spending a fortune on premium beauty products. Buy a nice body cream – you can get amazing ones in local pharmacies, supermarkets and pound shops – and rub it in after you have a bath. Tell your body how much you appreciate it as you're doing it. Your body has done so much for you over the years and now it's time for you to start taking care of it right back. Just that action alone will help to begin a change in attitude towards it.

Always remember to give yourself plenty of TLC. Run a bath at the end of the day and add a couple of drops of peppermint or tea tree oil. Have a long soak, rub in your cream and then get into bed. That is your end-of-day reward from now on, not a Mars bar.

YOU CAN DEAL WITH NEGATIVE THOUGHTS

You are stronger than you know. You're going to be breaking old patterns that put you where you are today, and that will be hard. I've never once said it would be easy. But it's going to be *worth it*! You've got this. Tell that whispering monkey on your back to bugger off. You're in charge now.

Negative thought processes may have been with you for many years, and until you start writing everything down you may not even realize how strong they were. But now you are in control.

EMBRACE TIREDNESS

Sometimes I get to the end of the day and I'm so tired all I want to do is snuggle up in bed and get a good night's sleep. I love that, because I sleep so well these days. My sleeping used to be erratic at times. But now I am so physically worn out, my head barely touches the pillow before I'm out like a light, and it's wonderful.

Don't worry about being tired, and don't fight it. If you need to have an early night, do it. You'll thank yourself in the long run, because you're learning new habits that will last a lifetime. By allowing your body to properly rest when it needs to, you're letting it know that it's being taken care of. If you look after your body, it will look after you.

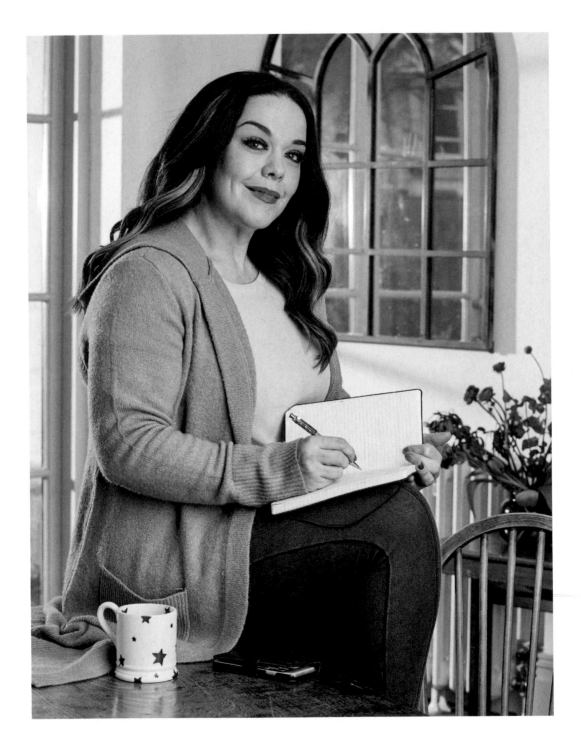

YOUR HONESTY DIARY IS STILL AN ESSENTIAL

I talked a lot about keeping an Honesty Diary in my previous book, and that's for a very good reason. My friends laugh at me because I've always got at least three journals on the go. One is a regular diary, so I know exactly what I'm supposed to be doing and when. Another is for work, so I can make notes on characters I'm playing or jot down ideas for roles or projects I'd like to do. And the third one is my Honesty Diary, which is an utter essential for me these days.

In fact, if anyone asks me what I recommend as the first step to take when embarking on a lifestyle overhaul like mine, it isn't to chuck out all the junk foods in your kitchen or buy a pair of trainers, it is to start an Honesty Diary in which you can document every single step of your journey.

Three years ago, when I first decided to put down the wine and family-sized trifle, I picked up a journal and I began writing. I've always kept a diary, and it made total sense to chart every step of the new journey I was embarking on so I could quickly work out where I was going wrong, and where I was going right. I wrote down how I felt, why I wanted to lose weight and how I planned to do it. Sometimes I wrote down just a few lines when they popped into my head, and other times I'd start writing and suddenly realize that two hours had gone by.

I charted the good stuff and the bad. The highlights and the low points. I wrote down everything I ate, so there was no hiding from it, and I wrote how I felt after each meal. I documented when I was getting cravings and what foods they were for, as well as how I was feeling when those pangs kicked in. When I felt tempted by crisps, I jotted it down, including what was going on to make me crave them, and I noted how I imagined I would feel if I gave in to those cravings. I learned so much about myself in such a short space of time. In the first few weeks alone I soon noticed patterns emerging and I realized how reliant I'd become on food as a sticking plaster.

For instance, if I was feeling stressed or upset I would want to comfort myself with stodge. I remember having this overwhelming desire for cake on one occasion in the early days of my weight loss. My period was due, I was feeling a little bit low and I wanted a quick fix. I could easily have walked into the nearest bakery and indulged. After all, who was going to stop me? But in the end, it was me who stopped me.

I wrote 'CAKE' in my diary in big letters. Underneath I wrote all the reasons why I wanted it: for comfort, as a reward for having been healthy for a couple of weeks, and just because I really, really liked cake! Then I wrote down the consequences if I caved in, which included feeling tired and bloated afterwards, and the fact it would probably kick off sugar cravings for a few days and throw my regime out of whack. Was it worth it? When I looked at the pros and cons there on paper in front of me, I could instantly see the answer was no. And giving myself five minutes to really consider it showed me that. By writing down everything that was going round in my head I could reason with those feelings, instead of pushing them down with junk food.

Getting things out of my head and into my diary freed me up from all the negative thought patterns that had been circling my mind like a merry-go-round. And I'd really like you to do the same.

In case you've not read my *Honesty Diet*, I'll explain again here how I like to structure my Honesty Diary. It's served me so well that I still do it exactly the same to this day.

Every day I wrote down:

- what time I ate
- what I ate
- why I ate it
- how it made me feel

Copy the grid opposite into your Honesty Diary or simply photocopy it lots of times, then get ready to start filling it in each day.

I still write in my diary each night before I go to bed – sometimes a lot and sometimes a little – so I don't have anything swirling around my mind while I'm trying to sleep. As well as noting down all the things I've eaten or drunk throughout the day, I also write down anything I've done that's made me feel proud/annoyed/happy, etc., what I hope to do tomorrow, and sometimes even longer-term plans for the future.

DATE	TIME	WHAT?	WHY?	HOW DID I FEEL?
BREAKFAST				
LUNCH				
DINNER				
SNACKS				
SUMMARY OF THE DAY				

CHALLENGE YOUR BLOCKAGES

Any time you feel like it, it can be very helpful to write down a really honest critique of yourself. Not to give yourself a hard time, but to make yourself aware of blockages. Jot down the things that are bothering you about yourself in that moment, or the things you're finding tricky, and then underneath write down what you think the solution might be. For instance:

- I feel lazy and sluggish:
  I'm going to get up and go for a walk tomorrow, even if I need to take it slowly.

- I'm not feeling very motivated with exercise at the moment:
  I'm going to have loads of fun putting together a new playlist of my favourite upbeat songs to help get me excited about working out.

- I'm still eating too much sugar:
  I'm going to eat a little bit less sugar tomorrow, and even less the day after, then slowly wean myself off it.

Every day, read your answers out loud to yourself five times and really absorb what you've written. If you say it often enough, you'll soon start to believe it.

You've just created your own positive affirmations!

By saying these affirmations out loud, you're telling yourself and your subconscious that you're ready to change. There is no limit to how many you can have or what they can be about. And they don't all have to be things you want to improve or change. Some can also be reminders of good things you've already got in your life. If you think your best asset is, say, your hair? Remind yourself! Write out a positive affirmation that says 'I have fabulous hair!' Have you helped someone through a tricky situation recently? Be proud of it with an 'I am a kind and empathetic person!' affirmation taped to your wall.

It's great to make these affirmations big and hard to miss, so I recommend using coloured markers to write your statements on big sheets of paper, or type them up and print them out. Stick them up on the wall, or pop them in a special Happiness Folder and put them near your bed to read through each morning. As long as your statements are positive they're allowed in your Happiness Folder or your Honesty Diary.

GET GRATEFUL

One of the things that has been life-changing for me is taking time to be grateful for what I have, and every day I include a gratitude list in my Honesty Diary. Sometimes I have to dig pretty deep, but when I put my mind to it there is always so much to be thankful for – even if it's just that someone smiled at me in the street, the sun is shining, or the fact I have a comfortable bed to sleep in. Those are all incredible things. Look for things to be thankful for on a daily basis and you will start to do it automatically after a while.

My friend Flossie and I often send each other lists of things we're happy about, and it's such a great reminder of how lucky we are. Why not start a Facebook or WhatsApp group with some mates so you can message each other a little list of wonderful things each day? You'll be surprised at how much of a difference it can make, and it's so nice to hear other people's uplifting messages too. Have a rule that you are only allowed to share positive things in that particular group. I bet you, if one of your friends is having a bad day it will cheer them up.

'Count your blessings' is one of the oldest sayings around, and it's been with us for so long because it's true, and it works. Make it a daily habit and you will start to look at life differently.

BE A VISIONARY

When I first read about vision boards several years ago, I thought they sounded a bit like a dodgy secondary school art project. But then I realized that they're basically like a real-life version of Pinterest, which I love.

The idea of a vision board is to gather together a collection of images that reflect your intentions and will help to make them feel real. These could be pictures cut out of magazines and newspapers, or printed off from the internet, and stuck to a giant board so you can look at it each day and be reminded of what you're aiming for. You could include:

- pictures of clothes you love, if you want to overhaul your wardrobe

- a picture of someone meditating, if you crave peace

- places you'd love to visit, even if you're just an armchair traveller for now

- a medal, if you're planning on running a 5k or even a marathon one day (hey, it could happen!)

You could also include positive phrases you identify with, and photos of people you admire or find inspirational. You can basically add anything you like that makes you feel positive, happy and inspired There's something about sourcing and cutting out inspirational pictures that helps bring your goals and ambitions to life. And it's a fun thing to do with kids, so you can get them involved too.

CHANGE YOUR MIND

Another brilliant thing to do (go with me on this one!) is to get yourself a whiteboard or a chalkboard and write 'I love me' on it. Look at it every day, and also look in the mirror and tell yourself out loud that you love yourself. You can even recount the reasons why or repeat your affirmations. It may sound a bit hokey, but believe me, it works!

You may be desperate for someone to say you look like you've lost weight or that your skin is glowing, but you can't expect other people to build you up. You have to do it for yourself. If you've started the day by telling yourself how amazing you are, you won't crave other people's compliments quite so much. You'll already be carrying your own self-approval around with you and wearing it with honour.

MINIMIZE YOUR LIFE

When I first decided I was going to lose weight, decluttering myself and my life was one of the best things I could have done. It created space around me and in my head, and it meant I wasn't distracted by the trivial things in life. What do I mean by decluttering? I mean getting rid of things you don't need any more, and hanging on to moments and memories rather than objects.

Clearing out my home and donating all the stuff I no longer wanted to charity was a huge boost. The amount of 'things' I had collected over the years as a security blanket felt overwhelming. I honestly felt like I was clearing out my mind while I was clearing clutter from my life. The less 'stuff' I had, such as clothes and homeware, the freer I felt. And it also benefited other people – so, happy days all round.

I also started saying no to things I didn't want to do. It took a bit of practice, because the people-pleaser in me wanted to do everything that was expected of me, but I realized that if I was going to take this weight-loss thing seriously I needed time and space to do it. I had always kept myself so busy I didn't have any time left for me. That was partly because I didn't want to face up to my issues, and partly because I'd never learned to stand up for myself. Add in hangovers, which are the ultimate time-waster, and there wasn't space in any given day to cook fresh food or squeeze in exercise. Something had to give.

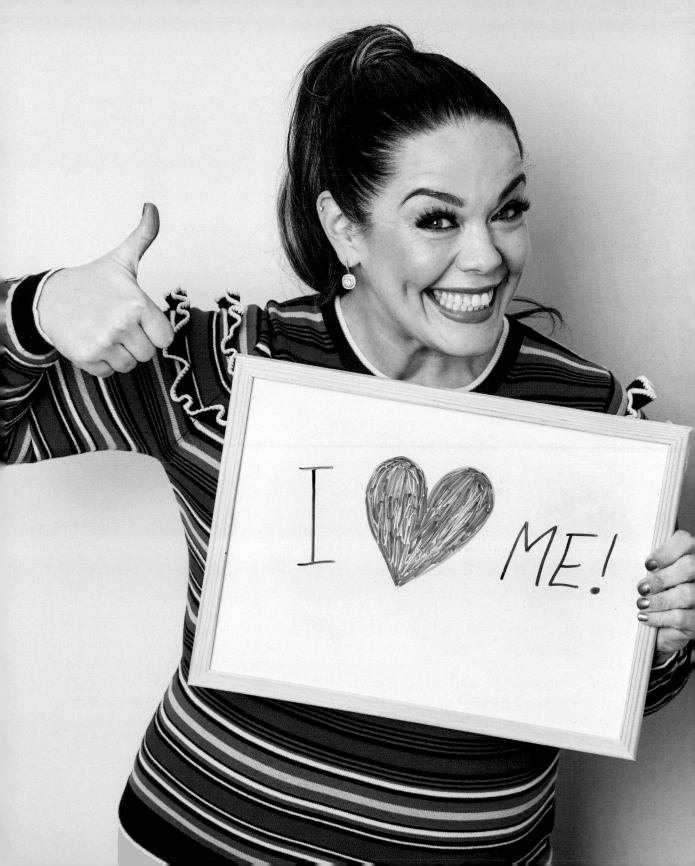

Once I started scheduling workouts in my diary, I found it easier to turn down other invitations because my exercise became more of a priority, and I didn't want to sacrifice it. I put myself first for a change. It took a long time for me to accept that it's not selfish, it's self-preservation. It goes back to that great analogy: you must put on your own oxygen mask on a plane before you can help anyone else put on theirs. You must take care of yourself first, otherwise you'll end up angry, tired and resentful and no use to anyone. You are every bit as important as other people.

TAKE TIME OUT

Time on your own is so important. I have a wonderful relationship with my partner, Al, but I still like to have 'my' time and 'my' space. I'm lucky enough to have an office in my house. When I need some space to write my journal or do some meditation I'll go in there. It's my sanctuary.

Find yourself some space, even if you have to lock the door of your bathroom to hide away and relax. Just do it! And remember that parents often get pushed to the back of the queue when it comes to self-care. They're so busy looking after others and making sure the kids are eating well and being entertained, they forget to look after themselves. If you're a parent, make a conscious effort not to fall into this trap.

GET A DIET BUDDY

I've talked before about how important it is to have an Honesty Buddy: someone who will always tell you the truth and who you can turn to when things get tough. How about getting a Diet Buddy too? That way you've got someone who can empathize with everything you're going through and spur you on if you're feeling disheartened. Support is my favourite dish!

If you don't have a friend or family member who could be your Diet Buddy, perhaps you could find someone online. I've met so many amazing people via my Facebook page, and they've all got the same goal: to lose weight and feel great. You could pop on to my page, have a look through the comments and posts, and if there's someone you identify with, perhaps drop them a message to see if they fancy partnering up and chatting about your goals. You can chart each other's progress and share recipe ideas, and you'll also be accountable to someone else, which is brilliant as it can help make you more committed. If you don't always feel like you can be totally honest with a friend, you can be completely honest with a stranger. We did the same thing for ITV's *Baggy Body Club*, and it worked so well. We were all going through similar experiences with our surgery and were able to get support and understanding whenever we needed it.

I remember talking to some friends about the pain I felt during a zumba class after my surgery. They did sympathize, but I couldn't help thinking, 'I'm not sure you truly understand how awful and painful it feels.' Then I spoke to Amanda from *The Baggy Body Club* and I could tell from her face that she got it exactly, because she'd been there too. If you look in the right place you will always find people who are going through the same things as you.

REMEMBER YOU'RE HUMAN

It's okay to have bad days. We're not perfect, and it's a bloody relief when you realize you never will be, and you don't have to be. We're human, we're not robots. Besides, even the most advanced computers have glitches every now and again. Once we accept that we're going to go through tricky times, life becomes easier to deal with. And once we have the tools to cope with those times, it becomes even better. It's okay to feel crap occasionally. Really! (Reread 'Crying is good', on page 15.)

SPOIL YOURSELF

I'm not suggesting that you go on an expensive shopping spree, because that's not sensible or necessary. Just buying yourself something small (perhaps a new hand cream), or setting some time aside to paint your toenails or read a book, helps remind you to care about yourself. Your rewards are no longer edible, remember. Discover the other things you love. For instance, I adore bath bombs. If I want to really treat myself I'll get one from Lush, but I'm just as happy with the ones from the pound shop. Once you start treating yourself to little things and making small changes, it will have a domino effect.

If you're giving up wine, cigarettes, junk food – or all three – the likelihood is you will find yourself saving money. So why not reinvest that spare cash in the most important thing in the world – you? You could put a fiver aside each week and treat yourself to something special at the end of the month. Like I said, we're not talking grand gestures here. Bath oil, body cream, a new journal and a sparkly pen are all you need for a wonderful, self-indulgent evening.

Another fantastic way to use that extra money could be on a personal trainer, even if it's just a one-off, or once every month or two. They can write you out a personalized plan based on your goals so, even if you never manage to have another session with them again, it's still money well spent.

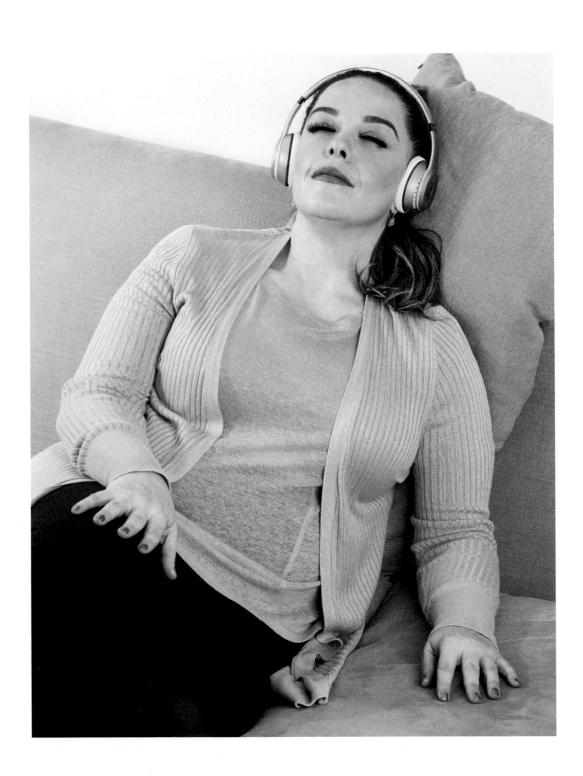

YOUR SELF-CARE CHECKLIST

It is a 'Lisa law' that you must do one of these kind things for yourself each day. And if you want to show yourself even more love, do a few of them:

- Ten minutes of deep breathing

- Ten minutes of stretching

- Cook a lovely healthy meal for yourself

- Have a long soak in the bath

- Read a book in peace

- Take yourself out for a coffee

- Go for a walk and appreciate the things around you, even if you just saunter around the block

- Look at photos from your childhood, or of family and friends

- Write a gratitude list

- Watch a meditation video on YouTube

- Give yourself a cuddle: literally, lie on your bed, wrap your arms around yourself and tell yourself how wonderful you are

- Watch an episode of your favourite show

- Browse online for fabulous clothes you're going to buy once you reach your dream size

- Phone a close friend for a chat

- Create a new vision board (see page 25), or copy some inspirational quotes into your Honesty Diary – see the next page for ideas!

FIND INSPIRATION

Talking of inspirational quotes, here are some of my favourites:

I am thankful for those difficult people in my life.
They have shown me exactly who I do not want to be.

Ninety-nine per cent of the things you worry
about never happen.

Many people have told me that I've changed. The truth
is I've just finally found myself.

If you want to change the fruits, you first have to
change the roots. To change the visible, first you have
to change the invisible. (T. Harv Eker)

People who shine from within don't need the spotlight.

If you can learn from the worst times of your life, you'll be
ready to go into the best times of your life.

Karma's only a bitch if you are.

Don't let the fear of what could happen
make nothing happen.

Before you assume, learn the facts. Before you judge, understand why. Before you hurt someone, feel. Before you speak, think.

The most valuable lessons aren't taught. They're experienced.

When you try to control everything, you enjoy nothing. Sometimes you just need to relax, breathe, let go and live in the moment.

You are strong when you know your weaknesses. You are beautiful when you appreciate your flaws. You are wise when you learn from your mistakes.

Yesterday is history. Tomorrow is a mystery. Today is a gift. That's why it is called the present.

If you are depressed, you are living in the past. If you are anxious, you are living in the future. If you are at peace, you are living in the present.

The day you realize you are superior to no one is when you realize that no one is superior to you.

WEAR IT WELL

My style has changed so much since I've lost weight and these days I absolutely love clothes. I particularly enjoy wearing colours and prints, and I now wear things that actually fit me. I get excited about what I can wear every single day.

In the old days I was very guilty of comfort shopping. Because I didn't feel particularly good in anything, I used to buy loads of clothes in the hope they would magically make me feel better. I'd grab shapeless things in my size even if I wasn't sure I even liked them, because finding something that would actually fit was my main priority. I was too embarrassed to try things on in changing rooms, so I'd usually buy them and take them home to try on in private. If they didn't fit, I rarely took things back because I was so worried about what the shop assistants might think. I wasted such a lot of money that way.

Some of my old dresses could have been repurposed as play tents for my nephews. The dress I wore when I was best woman for my brother Liam is hilarious. It's gigantic! I went through so much trauma searching for something that was smart, pretty and in my size. I wanted to look like the bee's knees for my brother on his special day and instead I was bursting out of the only dress I found that was suitable.

You could fit seven of me into that dress these days. I've kept it as a healthy reminder of where I used to be. I've only kept about nine or ten things from my bigger days because I wanted to wave goodbye to obese Lisa for good, but I think it's nice to keep the clothes that hold special memories, even if I didn't feel particularly attractive in them.

I still make style mistakes, and that's okay! I wore a beautiful maroon velour dress on *Loose Women* last year and for some reason it did not suit me at all. It didn't help that my hair looked like a giant doughnut on top of my head. My dad called me up afterwards and said, 'Lisa, what were you wearing? You looked massive.' Can I just say, in his defence, my dad and I are very honest with each other! And he was right. I did not dress for my shape that day.

Clothes are such a big deal to me now. I used to wear what I had to, but now I wear what I *want* to. These days I can choose things purely because they're gorgeous, and not just because of how much of my body they're going to cover up. And as for sexy underwear, that was something I never, ever wore! These days I adore wearing beautiful feminine sets, the silkier the better!

I can almost guarantee that as you lose weight your taste in clothes will change. You'll look at fashion differently. You'll notice styles you hadn't allowed yourself to see before because you were too afraid they wouldn't suit you. You will want to dress your new body in gorgeous things. You may buy your first pair of skinny jeans or start embracing colour. Take it from me, it's a really exciting time!

I've learned a fair few things from the stylists on shows I've worked on, both before and after my weight loss, and even more so while designing my own clothing range (Just Be You by Lisa Riley). These are the tips that really stood out for me:

- Don't wear clothes that are too big for you. If you're wearing a tent as a dress you're only going to look larger. You need to flatter and elongate your body by wearing things that fit.

- Don't wear clothes that are too small either. No one sees the size label in the back of your clothes but everyone sees what you look like when you're wearing them, and squeezing yourself into a size 16 when you're a 20 is not a good idea. If in doubt, go up a size or two and cut the label out if it really bothers you.

- Avoid a cropped trouser if you're a size 16 or above because they shorten your legs and therefore make you look bigger.

- Softly draped clothes are so much more sympathetic than smock styles. If clothes fall nicely they will flatter rather than enlarge you.

- Wrap-around dresses are every curvy girl's go-to. They accentuate your waist and give you curves, as well as making you look slimmer!

- Enjoy your good bumps and cover up your questionable ones.

- Try new styles and step out of your fashion comfort zone. It's like I say to my nephew Joshua about his food: try it, you might like it!

CHAPTER 2

My Failsafe Diet Rules

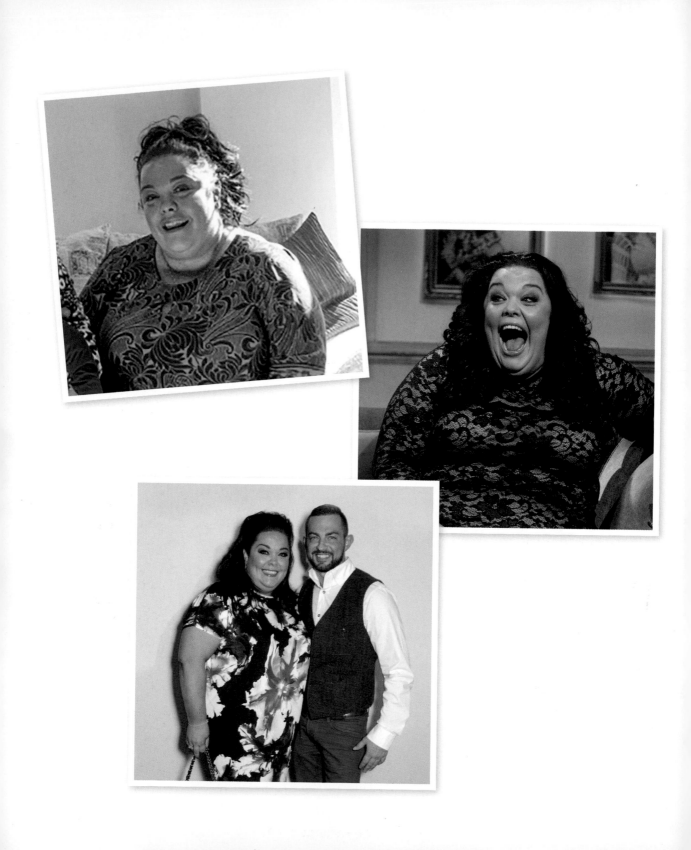

I didn't ever delude myself that by getting slimmer my life would suddenly be perfect. Everyone has their struggles, but it's bloody great that worrying about being able to fit into a seat on an aeroplane is no longer one of mine. The bottom line is that I did all of this for me and no one else. And you must do it for *you*. I didn't lose weight to impress people or to feel accepted – I've always been confident about who I am as a person, even when I was big – I did it because I wanted to wake up every morning feeling happy and full of energy. That, and helping other people, are still my main motivators. I love seeing people transform their bodies and become healthier and happier.

Such as Ruth, thirty-six, who followed the advice from my last book:

'Lisa's Honesty Diet helped me to get my head in the game and reassess what I want and need when it comes to food. Was I hungry sometimes while I did it? Yes, but it was so worth it and helped to reframe my thinking around food. My palate has changed since I did the kick-start plan, and I know it sounds crazy, but I do find myself craving healthy foods rather than sugar. A banana or raisins are enough for me now. In fact, they've become a treat, and I'm amazed about that. Now I only eat when I'm hungry, which sounds so obvious, but the book and kick-start plan taught me that I didn't need to eat as much as I had been. I never thought I would get to that point. My eating pendulum had swung way too far in the wrong direction, but now it's come back to the middle. I dropped two dress sizes in seven weeks and I'm excited about dropping more.'

The Timehop app is still another massive motivator for me. It shows me pictures of how I looked on the same day in previous years. When I see 'me times two' staring back in pictures from several years ago, I get this overwhelming sense of relief that I never have to be in that place again.

When I look back at how I looked then, it instantly reminds me of how I felt. I was tired all the time, I was sluggish, and although I did a very good job of pretending I was happy, it was horrible being the one that dominated all the photos of me with my mates purely because I was so much bigger than all of them. I look as if someone has stuck a pump in my mouth and inflated me. Sometimes when I look at old photos now, I barely even recognize myself.

I still stop and ask myself how I got so big. Well, I know the logistics of how I did – because of the amount of crap I used to eat – but what's confusing for me is how I allowed it to happen. Why didn't I stop when things got out of control?

I know now that it was self-preservation that stopped me facing up to it. Subconsciously I knew that it was going to hurt when I eventually admitted that I didn't look and feel like I really wanted to. It was also hard to face up to the fact that I was shockingly unhealthy and felt sluggish most of the time. It was so much easier to carry on playing the character that everyone expected me to be, rather than change. Denial may be an unhappy place to be, but it's safe.

I was very good at self-narrating. If I ever felt bad about how I looked, a voice would instantly kick in that said, 'Don't worry about it, Lisa. This is just how you're supposed to be. This is your path.' And that made me feel comfortable. I guess in the same way as I now tell myself every day that I want to feel good – and I know I deserve to – 'fat me' told myself every day that I was fine as I was. Was I heck!

It's hard to change your life but, my God, it's fabulous on so many levels when you do. I remind myself every day of how I used to feel, and that's what pushes me on. The new me is so comfortable with myself. Maybe a little too much sometimes! I really don't mind if people walk in when I'm getting changed backstage at a show. I think I've shocked a few people in recent times . . .

These days when I get out of the shower naked, with my hair in a towel, I don't mind seeing myself in a mirror. In fact, I'm so thrilled that I often can't stop looking! Don't get me wrong, I don't feel amazing or sexy every day. I have rubbish days just like everyone, and days when I worry that the weight will go back on. I can slip back into my old self-critical ways pretty easily, and I need to have a stern word with myself to get my head back into the right place. When I'm aware I'm being stupid, I'll write down everything I'm feeling and work through it. Life isn't about skipping through cornfields every day, and it can be tough. But if you have self-awareness and you're willing to work at it, you really can change how you think.

It's like that saying 'A dog is for life, not just for Christmas.' Healthy eating and a good mindset aren't just for while you're on a diet, they should be for life. If you've hopped on and off diets for years and they haven't worked for you, that's because you've got to change your thinking and face up to the fact that you can't eat well for just a few months and then go back to eating tubs of ice cream in front of the TV every night. Funnily enough, you won't keep the weight off if you do that. This is about long-term change.

There are lots of times when I catch myself and cannot believe how different things are for me now. I spoke in my previous book about how I once cried with happiness on a plane after I lost weight because I no longer needed an extender for my seat belt, and people didn't look panicked when they realized they'd have to sit next to me.

I had another one of those amazing moments last year. I was flying back from a work trip to America and I got upgraded, which was incredible. The last time I'd flown First Class had been years before, when I went away with a couple of friends and was so excited about the prospect of having a bed to lie down in and a TV to watch. I thought it was going to be such a fun journey, but when I saw the seat I knew immediately that there was no way I was going to be able to lie down in it. I would have been wedged in really uncomfortably. My two friends both snuggled up, watching their telly or sleeping, but I sat bolt upright, feeling very squashed even in First Class, which is meant to be roomy. It was so depressing.

This time was so different. As soon as I boarded the plane I immediately clicked my seat down into a bed, and as I lay there with the duvet wrapped around me, with so much room on either side, tears started rolling down my cheeks. That was one of the moments when I thought, 'It's all been worth it.' Every difficult moment, every scar and every negative comment that had ever been aimed at me felt like a drop in the ocean. Those moments of realization are the ones I cherish most, which is why I love sharing them.

Ask yourself the question:

Do you want to be happy in your skin for the rest of your life?

If you do, you have to put the work in. It will be so worth it. I promise.

I'm learning more and more about myself, and about health and fitness, every day, and I want to share the things that have kept me on track. These rules, and the ones I wrote about in my *Honesty Diet*, are for your head as well as your body. They are proper game changers.

BE REALISTIC

When I have a bad day I tell myself that I'm human and I'm a size 12, and I'm realistic about that. I do not have the body shape to be a size 8, and nor would I want to be that small. I would definitely get a lollipop head. I'm not delusional and I know my limits. I didn't kid myself that when I slimmed down I would suddenly look like Jennifer Lopez, because the only person in the world who looks like that is Jennifer Lopez. And the only person in the world who looks like me is me, and the only person in the world who looks like you is you. (Not that I'd say no to having a bottom like J-Lo's!)

Work with your natural shape and make that the best it can be, whether you're supposed to be long and lean or petite and curvy. If you're going to change your body for life then you need to be honest with yourself. I do a lot of boxing, so I have muscles in my upper back that can make me look quite broad, and I'm never going to be a slip of a thing. No one is ever going to be scared I'll fall through the gap in a drain, because I have a strong body. It's toned and muscular now, and that's what I love. I adore that athletic, fit look, and that's what I aspire to. I love Davina McCall's definition, and that's the next level of where I want to be. I started singing that Shania Twain song 'Man, I Feel Like a Woman' the other day, because I do. I always admired Drew Barrymore's body shape because she was toned but curvy, and she looked gorgeous and womanly, and now I feel like that too.

There is no such thing as being the right shape. Just YOUR right shape.

Fashions change, and not just for clothes and decor, but for bodies too. Years ago it was considered to be a flaw if you had a big bum. Now, thanks to the likes of the Kardashians and J-Lo, they're all the rage. In the sixties thin eyebrows were high fashion, and now it's all about having big bushy ones. How are we ever supposed to feel good enough, or like we fit in, when the goalposts keep moving? What's 'right' in the fashion magazines one day might not be right the next, but being happy with who we are will always be on-trend.

TAKE YOUR TIME

When I set out on this journey I told myself that Rome wasn't built in a day. I knew I could get to where I wanted, but it had to be one step at a time. The problem is that we all want to rush from the start to the finish but we don't want to do the bits in between, which are essential. That's why crash diets don't work. You'll get to the finish line in record time. But before you know it you'll be back on the starting line, because the weight will pile back on so quickly. If you do the important bits slowly and carefully you won't have to take any steps back, because your body will adjust and the weight will naturally stay off. It's about learning how to eat properly, eat well and change old patterns. That doesn't happen overnight. But once you've got those new teachings locked in your head, they're not going anywhere. It's absolutely worth taking that extra time.

It took me over two years to lose all my weight. Could I have lost it more quickly if I'd starved myself or had a gastric band fitted? Probably. But I wouldn't have learned a hundredth of what I've ended up learning. I've now got tools for life that will serve me well forever. This is for always, so it has to be gradual. Do everything at your own pace. If you take things slowly you'll achieve lasting change.

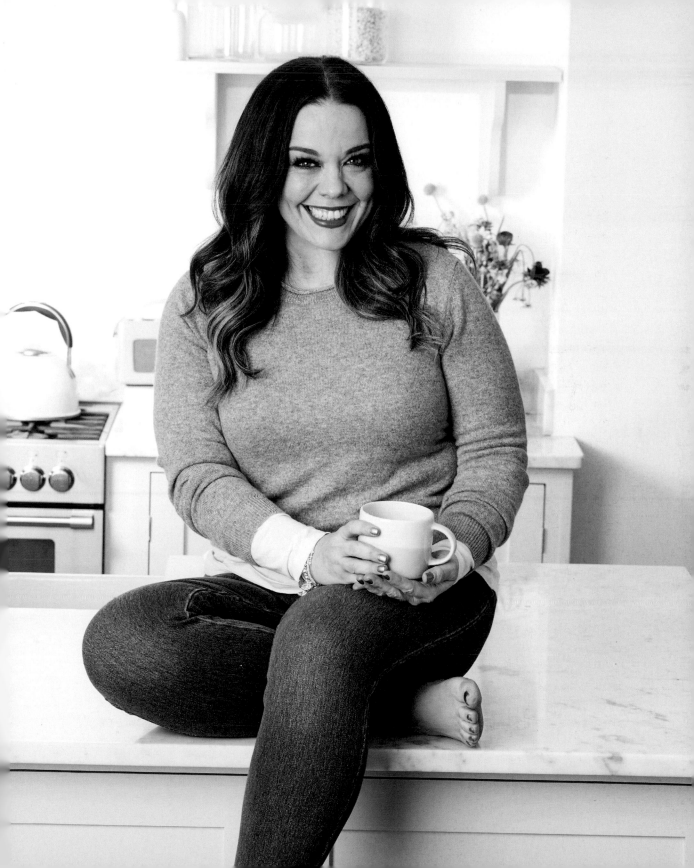

By taking things slowly you're giving your body a chance to catch up and understand what's going on rather than sending it into panic mode. We're changing things for life here, so it's worth being patient.

You do not have to starve yourself! The surprising thing is that you can actually eat quite a lot on a diet; you just have to eat the right things. It really is that simple. If you try and live on two KitKats a day you may lose weight quickly, but your body won't know what's hit it. The minute you start eating normally again – and I'm sorry to break it to you but existing on two KitKats isn't normal – your body is going to suck up every single bit of food you put into it and . . . boom! However, if you get your body into a routine and you nourish it and look after it, it will look after you.

Jockeys can't win the Grand National unless they jump over each hurdle that's in their way, and weight loss is exactly the same. You will come up against hurdles, just like you do in everyday life, whether it's your weight plateauing or being tempted by canapés and wine at a party. Some of those hurdles you will be able to fly over, while others will be much harder to negotiate. But when you've jumped them once, you'll have the confidence to know you can do it again, and that is the best feeling.

LOOK AT WHAT YOU HAVE GOT, NOT WHAT YOU HAVEN'T

We are all very good at focusing on what we haven't got, or what we haven't done, rather than what we have. I look at my legs and think, 'My scars look bad today.' But what I should be thinking is, 'Wow, look at the muscles I've got in my thighs!' I don't always do that, and I'm working on it. I pride myself on not judging people, but I still judge myself. That's something that's getting better over time. Acceptance is such a key element in making changes.

I was in Mykonos on holiday last year. I was wearing this beautiful swimsuit that a few years ago I could never have dreamed of wearing, and I was lying there on the sun lounger picking holes in my appearance. The funny thing is, I didn't do that when I was bigger. I was in such denial – my body felt like an impossible thing to tackle – so I told myself that's just the way I was. I felt overwhelmed by how large I was, and didn't think I could ever look any better, so I didn't even try. I remember looking in the mirror on that holiday last year and thinking, 'I wish my calves were more defined.' I mean, seriously, three years ago I don't think I even knew calves could be defined.

Once I started to lose weight I quickly began to put a lot more pressure on myself. Now, if I'm giving myself a hard time about something, I will sit down and work out why by writing it down. Sometimes it's just because I'm not feeling great and I'm projecting those feelings on to my body. But once it's down on paper, and I can understand it more, it goes away so much quicker. I try to turn every negative into a positive. If I'm thinking, 'My bra cupcake is really bothering me today,' I tell myself how toned my bum looks or remind myself that I'm wearing a pair of size 12 trousers.

SCALES = FAILS

I made a pretty big deal of this in my previous book and it's making a comeback because it's so important. Stop weighing yourself! I know that the scales still do not work for me. If I step on them when I'm having a crap day they will not make me feel any better. In fact, if I've put on a few pounds it will totally demotivate me and make me miserable. Your weight can fluctuate so much, and even going to the toilet can make a difference, hence my mantra 'scales = fails'. Please don't do it to yourself!

You cannot hinge all of your self-esteem on whether you weigh two or three pounds more or less on one particular day. You're not a bad person if you're a bit more bloated on Tuesday than you were on Monday. That's why it's so important to like yourself. That way, if you do have a bad body day you're less likely to panic and start comfort eating. If you have one of those days, write down all the things you like about yourself – whether it's your eyebrows, or the fact that you're kind, or you're a great friend. Your character traits are every bit as important as whether or not you look good in skinny jeans. They go hand in hand with feeling amazing.

ASK FOR HELP

Always ask for help when you're struggling. If I feel rubbish, the first thing I do is tell someone. I'll be honest about it with my partner, Al, and I think that's really important. Don't pretend everything is okay if it isn't. If you've found yourself an Honesty Buddy or Diet Buddy like I've suggested, someone you can be completely open with about your weight-loss goals and challenges, then they are a great person to confide in at times like this.

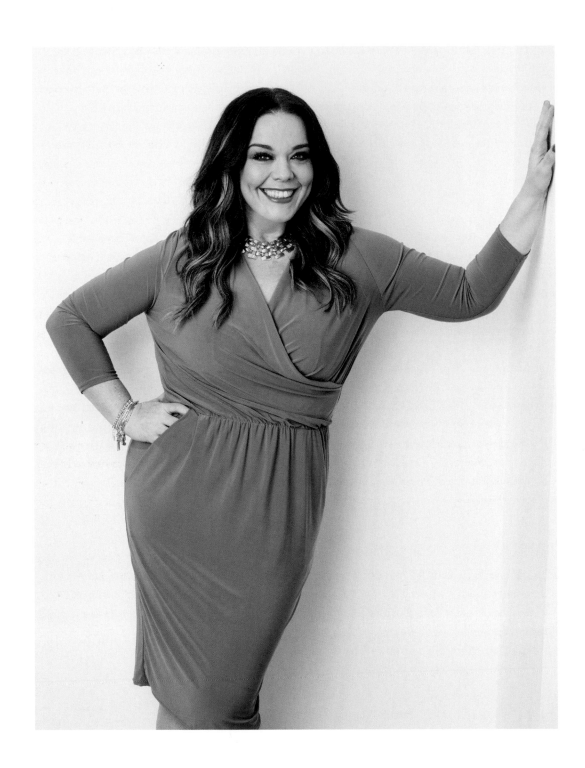

DON'T USE FOOD AS A COMFORT OR REWARD

I used to go and dive into a box of doughnuts if I was feeling bad, but now I'll go to an exercise class. I get much better results than I would do from a large packet of Mini Eggs!

You learn from a really young age that food is a reward and a comfort. I was quietened with chocolate when I was a child. My gran would give me a bar of something if she wanted me to settle down, and that stayed with me. You're told as a kid that if you're good you can have a treat, and you can bet that treat was never an apple or a handful of nuts. So no wonder when you feel rubbish you instantly reach for something stodgy or loaded with sugar to make you feel better. You're just repeating old patterns. You weren't born with a desire to stuff your face with bags of Kettle Chips or burgers if you're stressed, you learned it along the way. But the great thing about patterns is that you can break them.

We still reward ourselves as adults. Got a promotion at work? Let's roll out the wine and crisps! It's your birthday? Have a cake! Done a long workout? You deserve a muffin! No, you don't. Not if you want to lose that muffin top.

DON'T USE YOUR PERIOD AS AN EXCUSE

I know that periods can be a real trigger for women to eat. Not only do you often feel hungrier and crave comfort foods like bread and chocolate and cheese, but the time of the month can encourage a 'Sod it, I'm allowed' attitude. You might think, 'I feel big anyway, so I may as well eat.' Don't. It will pass. You know that your period will be over in a few days, and normal life will resume. You can get through it.

When I get like that, I eat bananas or apples dipped in peanut butter to tackle my sugar cravings. And water is your friend. It may feel counter-intuitive to drink fluids if you're suffering from water retention, but actually it will help your body to flush everything out. When I get period bloating and water retention, I find the best way for me to deal with that is to go swimming. It's gentle but it gets my body moving, and I always feel better afterwards.

PARK PERFECTION

I'm going to say something that might surprise you now: it's okay to make mistakes when you're dieting. It's okay to slip up, it's okay to get things wrong. Wobbles are normal. If you fall off the wagon, simply pick yourself up and look to the future. A little slip does not have to equal a slippery slope.

A woman messaged me on Twitter recently to confess that she'd been to her friend's house and ended up eating two cookies, and now she was annoyed with herself. I told her, don't be! Okay, you've done it, now get over it. We've all had moments like this. It's important not to give yourself a massively hard time, or you'll feel so miserable you'll probably end up eating two more packets. A blip is just that. Take a deep breath and get back on the right path.

AVOID OVEREATING

I know, I know – simple to say, hard to do. I explained in my *Honesty Diet* that I eat from bowls now instead of plates, and it really makes a difference to the amount I consume. I've gone from piling massive portions on to giant plates to having neat bowls of food. My brain has got used to it, and there is no way on earth I could go back to eating like I did before. I would feel so sick and uncomfortable.

I was with a friend in a restaurant recently and she ordered a BLT. The waitress asked if she wanted fries and she said no, because she wasn't that hungry. When the order came there was a big bowl of fries with it, but for some reason she didn't send them back. When the waitress walked away my friend said, 'Ooh, I shouldn't, but I will,' and she tucked into the chips. At one point she was so full she had to stop and take deep breaths before she could fit more in, but she ended up polishing off the lot. She probably didn't even realize how much she'd eaten; she'd switched off her guilt sensor and was eating mindlessly. I didn't say anything, and of course I have absolutely no right to judge, but it was interesting to observe. I can imagine her belly must have felt so uncomfortable. She didn't want those fries, she'd already made that clear, but she ate them anyway.

Five minutes later she said to me, 'I really don't want to go shopping now. I feel too fat.' Her self-esteem had taken a real kick in the teeth, right there. How are you supposed to feel good about your body if you're overloading it and then feeling full and uncomfortable? If you say, 'Hold the fries,' you have to mean it. Just because you didn't order them it doesn't mean they don't count!

The most valuable lessons aren't taught, they're experienced.!!

Even if you eat something without thinking about it, I'm afraid it will still have an impact on your weight. Maybe more so, because if you're eating mindlessly you won't even be aware of how much you're consuming. Back in the old days I could eat five bars of chocolate and then look in the bin and think, 'Where the hell did those wrappers come from?' I would barely remember eating them, let alone hiding the wrappers.

I do understand overeating because I've been there. I know it's a comfort thing. I've seen people do it when they're bored or lonely, and I used to be really guilty of it myself. But at its extreme it's a form of self-abuse, and I honestly know now that I had an addiction to food, and not good food. So my number one tip for avoiding overeating brings me neatly to my next rule.

SLOW DOWN!

It's something that's been said for years, and people roll their eyes because it's so simplistic, but eating slowly really does make a difference. Your brain takes a while to catch up with your stomach, so you may be full much sooner than you realize. Chew your food really well, and really taste each mouthful. When you start eating smaller portions, or stopping when you're full, your body begins to adapt. You won't be physically able to eat as much as you once did without feeling bloated and lethargic. And who wants to feel like that?

Some good tips are:

- Always try to sit down at a table to eat.
- Don't eat in front of the TV because it will distract you, and there's a higher risk you'll overeat. The same goes for your phone: nothing will happen on Facebook in the time it takes to eat your meal.
- Put down your knife and fork in between mouthfuls.
- Chew your food properly. I know that sounds ridiculous, but so many people don't – and your stomach doesn't have its own set of teeth, so it can't chew your meal again once it gets down there!
- Taste your food and enjoy every bit of it. Especially if you've cooked it yourself. Appreciate what a great job you've done, and allow yourself to experience all the different flavours.

Once you've nailed these things, you've nailed them forever. These are habits that you want to stay with you for the rest of your life. It really will make all the difference.

STOP FEELING GUILTY EVERY TIME YOU EAT

It's a simple fact that we must eat to live. Yes, we want to be mindful of what we're putting in our mouths but we do need to have three sensible, balanced, nutritious meals a day and not feel guilty about those. For anyone who has experienced a lifetime of dieting, it's likely they'll have restricted themselves to quite an extreme degree at some point. As a result, whenever they've come off their diet they've probably been left feeling bad every time they ate something.

Do people feel guilty when they drink water? No, because we must have fluids to stay alive. And there's no reason to feel guilty about eating either, because it's literally a life force. Yes, you need to make the right choices and consume foods that are good for your body, but don't ever give yourself a hard time about sitting down to an incredible salad, stir-fry or casserole. Your body needs that fuel and all the minerals, vitamins and goodness, and it will thank you for it. Dieting does not mean not eating.

YOUR BODY IS TOO CLEVER FOR YOU

Your body knows when you're eating too much, and it knows when you're eating too little. You can't outwit it. If you feed it too little, it will panic and you will feel weak and terrible. If you load it up with too much food, you will put on weight. It's not rocket science.

A friend of mine said to me recently that she'd had this amazing revelation to do with her diet and body, and it really struck a chord with me. She said that for so long she'd been annoyed with her body because she wasn't a toned size 10. Then one day she sat there and thought, 'Maybe that's because I eat too much crap, drink too much wine and don't do enough exercise.' And there it is, right there. That's the honest answer. Now she's started being honest with herself about the fact that she's been burying her head in the sand, and things are really starting to shift for her. I don't just mean the excess weight; I mean her attitude towards diet and exercise.

She was expecting to have a great body without putting in any of the work. If you want your nails to look nice you have to take care of them. That doesn't just magically happen on its own. It's the same with your body. It will support you and keep you as healthy as it possibly can, but if you're not taking care of it properly it's not going to look or behave exactly how you want it to.

DON'T FALL FOR DIET TRICKS

Just because a food packet says the words 'diet', 'slimline' or 'healthy' on it, it doesn't mean it is. Studies have shown that some regular biscuits have fewer calories and less sugar and fat than many of the ones you're told will help you lose weight. If in doubt, check packets thoroughly. All the information you need is right there. Look past the colourful packaging and the pictures of slim, smiling women who don't have a care in the world. Look at the facts! There is no guarantee of instant happiness waiting for you inside that packet, and you will not wake up tomorrow a size smaller if you eat a 'low-fat' biscuit.

I know it's hard. I know. Every time we walk into a supermarket we're being targeted. The aisles aren't organized in the way they are by chance. The brightly coloured fruit and vegetables are the first things we see because the nice displays put us in a good mood. How bizarre is that? It's also not a coincidence that the more expensive products are at eye level, while the cheaper ones get put on the bottom or top shelf so you have to search for them. Wine and crisps aren't placed close to each other by chance. Both are 'treat' items, so you're more likely to buy them together if they're in the next aisle.

You're fighting a losing battle. The smell of warm bread or chickens roasting is being pumped out to make you feel hungry so you buy more, and before you know it you're filling your basket with foods you didn't plan to buy. Stick to your list! We all love a bargain but three-for-two deals are a nightmare. If you only need one of something, only buy one. If you buy three, you'll eat three. Or you'll end up throwing two away when they go out of date. How many times have you seen 'Only at the bakery today!' signs offering you cheap cakes? We all fall for it. We panic and think we may never get a deal that good again. Here's the thing: the same deal will probably be available tomorrow and the day after and . . . You get my drift.

Don't get me started on the food by the till. Shops load up small snacks by the till that will trigger your 'f**k it' button. Have you noticed that they don't ever put TVs by the till? Of course they don't, because who goes and does their weekly shop and then gets to the till and thinks, 'Oh, while I'm here, I may as well get a new telly'? No one. But how many people think, 'Ooh, a Snickers. Well, it's only little, and it's right here. Might as well'? So many people. I see it all the time – I call them the 'last-minuters'. Those 'little' last-minute things can ruin your diet. It's a classic 'it'll be fine' moment.

If you had planned to buy that Snickers bar, you would have already gone to the chocolate aisle and got one. But you didn't, because you're trying to eat healthily. It's still equally as fattening, whether you meant to buy it or whether it was a last-minute decision.

When was the last time you saw piles of bananas or oranges while you were waiting to pay for your shopping? I know I haven't. It's always unhealthy foods, because supermarkets know they've got a captive audience. I know so many people who don't even make it out of a supermarket car park without eating something. Then, by the time they're home, the snack amnesia kicks in and they've forgotten it ever happened. They'll get to the end of the day and think they've done really well because they'll be in denial about the Twix they wolfed down while they were driving.

One way to counteract all the temptation of going to a supermarket is to get online deliveries. That way you will only order what you actually need, and it's impossible to do a last-minute panic grab!

I was in a newsagent's recently and when I paid for a magazine at the counter they asked me if I wanted to buy a massive bar of chocolate because it was on special offer. Erm, no? If I'd wanted to buy a huge bar of chocolate I would have picked it up and brought it to the counter with me.

Losing weight is, essentially, pretty simple.

I cannot say this enough times – the only diet that truly works is eating well, moving around more and changing your attitude towards food for life.

The thing about diets is that if one worked amazingly there wouldn't be hundreds of them. Every January we're offered a ton of new ways to lose weight that promise to be easier, more satisfying and quicker than ever before. Some of them will even try and tell you that you won't even realize you're on a diet. RUBBISH! If it really was that easy, wouldn't we all be effortlessly slim?

You can walk into a shop and spend £30 on some diet tea, but if you're still sitting down in front of the TV with a giant bar of chocolate every night that tea isn't going to make a blind bit of difference. And don't get me started on slimming tablets. Walk. Away. Aside from some of them being dangerous, taking tablets for a few months isn't going to change your mindset in the long term. Any weight you lose will be temporary, and you can't stay on pills for the rest of your life unless you're willing to seriously damage your body.

CHAPTER 3

The 8-day Kick-Start

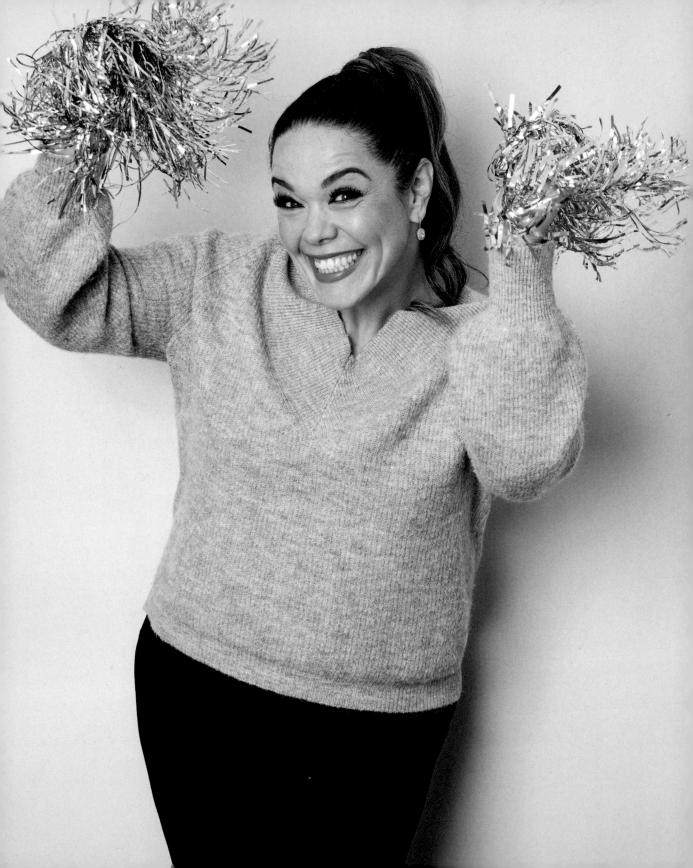

We're going to prepare for your new lifelong lifestyle with an 8-Day Kick-Start. It was one of the things people loved about my previous book, and many readers got in touch to share their success. So here's a whole new plan to get stuck into. I'm mixing things up a bit this time around, and as well as the daily food and exercise programme, I'm also incorporating mental well-being exercises for an even more comprehensive approach that will set you on the road to success.

If you've not followed a plan like this before, it may look a bit daunting at first glance. It's designed to produce some visible initial weight loss, because there's nothing more motivating than seeing changes in yourself, so this will help set you off in the right direction. You may find it tough, but remember, it's only eight days out of your life – long enough to get a result, but short enough that the finish line is always in sight. You will feel so proud of yourself once it's done and dusted. You'll have proved to yourself that you're strong enough to make a change, and that's a feeling you'll be able to keep hold of forever. Those eight days seem worth it now, don't they?

During this period you'll be eating less and doing more exercise than you're probably used to, so you may feel hungry and tired as your body adjusts. It's best to get plenty of sleep so that you have a chance to recover and re-energize before each day. If you experience any constipation, eat an apple or pear (with skin), a handful of berries or a side of broccoli with your lunch or dinner, as these all contain good amounts of fibre and will help get things moving again. Make sure to drink lots of water to stay hydrated throughout the plan. If you experience any headaches, water should also help to ease these. If you normally drink tea or coffee, switch to herbal tea or hot water with lemon. (Though if you regularly drink a lot of caffeine, I highly recommend you begin cutting down your intake in advance, else you may experience withdrawal headaches throughout the kick-start, which won't help put you in the right frame of mind for success.)

As well as following the meal plan, I would like you to aim for half an hour of exercise every day, ideally doing some form of cardio so you break a sweat. I know that might sound a lot, so if you need to split it up into a couple of smaller chunks, that's fine. And if you're new to exercise, you may need to start with less and gradually build up. But whatever you do, make sure you are challenging yourself, because the point here is to let your body know you mean business. Saying that, it's important to be sensible and take care of your body. Stay well hydrated, and if you ever feel dizzy or faint, stop exercising immediately and seek medical advice. The plan isn't meant to be easy, but it also shouldn't damage your health. Push yourself, but also look after yourself.

Talking of which, I'd also like you to do at least one thing each day from my self-care checklist on page 31. And don't forget to write in your Honesty Diary too, even if you only have time to write a few lines.

This Kick-Start will help you get your mind and body into the right zone for the next phase of the diet, which involves eating well for life. At the end of the eight days, please don't just revert to how you used to eat, or your hard work will simply go to waste! Instead, I'd like you to follow my failsafe diet rules (see Chapter 2) as well as applying my mindset and eating advice from the other parts of the book, while also continuing to exercise several times a week (see workout ideas pages 102–21) and cooking your way through my other healthy recipes on pages 127–247. Remember: if you eat better (i.e. healthy food in smaller portions), move more and apply some common sense, that excess weight will come off and stay off.

It's time to get going on the plan, so here are a few handy tips to make sure you get off to a great start:

- Start each day with hot water and lemon, which can either be freshly squeezed or out of a bottle, whichever you prefer. As well as giving your immune system a little boost, this will rehydrate you after sleep.

- Drink at least two litres of water a day to stay hydrated and keep you feeling fuller.

- Lunch is going to be your main meal of the day so your body has plenty of time to burn it off.

- Snacks aren't part of this plan I'm afraid – unless you're really struggling and on the verge of quitting. If that's truly the case, have a handful of almonds or grapes to help you through. Remember, it's only for eight days!

- If there are any meals you don't like, you can substitute them for one from another day, but it must be from the same time of day, i.e. you can swap one breakfast for another one, but not a breakfast for a lunch.

IMPORTANT: This diet is not suitable for pregnant or breastfeeding women, nor for children, teenagers, those with a history of eating disorders or anyone who is frail or unwell. You should consult with a doctor or healthcare professional before embarking on the plan to ensure you are in good health and to make sure it's the right choice for you, especially if you are on any kind of medication or treatment plan. It's always a good idea to get medical advice, particularly if you have a lot of weight to lose, in which case I also recommend you seek the guidance of a registered nutritionist if you can.

	BREAKFAST	LUNCH	DINNER
DAY 1	Hot water and lemon Two boiled eggs	Vegetable red Thai curry (p.149)	Fish stew (p.184)
DAY 2	Hot water and lemon Skinny omelette wrap (p.220)	Coconut chicken salad (p.178)	White bean and garlic soup (p.133)
DAY 3	Hot water and lemon Overnight chia oats with berries (p.212) (make enough for tomorrow too)	Italian-style chicken tray bake (p.146)	Celeriac and apple soup with chilli oatcakes (p.130)
DAY 4	Hot water and lemon Overnight chia oats with berries (p.212) (leftover portion from yesterday)	Grilled salmon and ratatouille (p.141)	All green soup (p.132)
DAY 5	Hot water and lemon Buckwheat porridge with orange and cinnamon (p.129)	Butter bean and chicken sausage stew (p.166)	Miso-roasted cod with pan-fried greens (p.167)
DAY 6	Hot water and lemon One poached egg with big handful of wilted spinach	Italian-style chicken tray bake (p.146)	Veggie noodle stir-fry (p.142)
DAY 7	Hot water and lemon Small bowl of fruit salad with low-fat Greek yoghurt	Spicy turkey and quinoa stuffed peppers (p.204)	Baked falafel salad (p.186)
DAY 8	Hot water and lemon Spinach, broccoli, kiwi and Greek yoghurt smoothie (p.216)	Chickpea and spinach curry (p.156)	Spicy poached chicken broth (p.174)

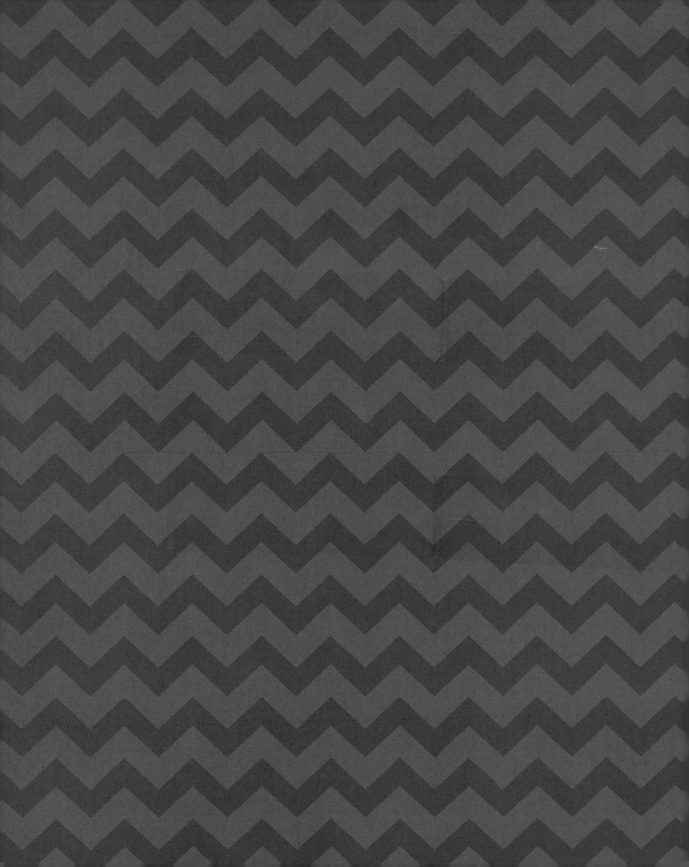

CHAPTER 4

Ask Lisa...

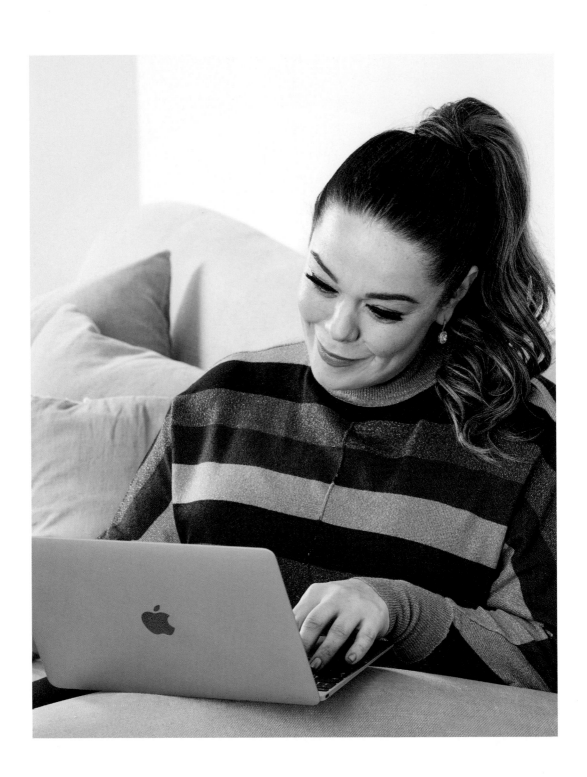

I get asked a lot of diet and fitness questions these days – mostly online, but sometimes even by people who stop me in the street – so I thought it would be useful to share my answers to the ones that crop up most often, in case you find yourself facing similar uncertainties and challenges.

DIETS MAKE ME FEEL TIRED. HOW DO I PERK MYSELF UP?

You may feel tired at the start, while your body is adjusting to a new regime, and initially it's just a case of riding it out. Your body will soon catch up. I went on a week-long boot camp recently and by day four I didn't want to get out of bed because my body was still several steps behind. But I made myself get up and crack on, and I soon got back into the swing of things. It's all about willpower and determination. You might think that I'm being tougher in this book, and perhaps I am, but I really want to help you make and see the changes.

If you're feeling tired, doing exercise will actually help you find more energy. It releases endorphins, which are a stimulant, so even if you go on an exercise bike for twenty minutes you will feel so much better. People say to me, 'If I'm tired, I want to lie on the sofa and recharge my batteries.' No! A class or a workout pumps you up and does the job much more effectively.

SHOULD I EXERCISE IF I'M ILL?

No, it's not a good idea to exercise when you're unwell. It will only make you more tired, so you need to give your body a rest. I tried to work out when I was ill once and my blood pressure plummeted. I saw stars, which is not at all good. I admitted defeat and went straight home to bed. The quicker you recover, the quicker you'll be able to get up and moving about again.

I KNOW I NEED TO LOSE WEIGHT BUT I JUST CAN'T GET INTO THE ZONE. WHERE AM I GOING WRONG?

Being vaguely aware of something and properly admitting it to yourself are two very different things. You might be aware that you are overweight and that you need to do something about it, but until you fully admit it to yourself it's unlikely you'll move on. The first step is admitting that you really do want to be slimmer and not continuing to tell yourself that you're fine as you are. That's the breakthrough moment, so be prepared that you may cry when you realize. I know I did.

The moment I knew I was ready to lose weight was when I stopped making jokes about myself. I also stopped justifying how much I was eating and how little I was exercising, and I stopped making excuses about why I couldn't lose weight. Instead, I got on and did it.

I'M GREAT AT STICKING TO THE PLAN DURING THE WEEK. BUT WHY DO I ALWAYS FALL OFF THE WAGON AT WEEKENDS?

Don't worry, this is really common. I think it's mentally harder if you work during the week, because you come to see the weekend as your time to relax, and people associate weekends with treating themselves. It's traditionally the time you go to the pub for a few drinks or get a takeaway, so I do understand that it can be tricky to stick to your diet. It's those old habits rearing their heads again. But the reality is that you've often got much more time to exercise at the weekends, especially if you find ways for your family to be involved. Go to swim club with the kids and nip into the gym while they're in their lesson, or also do some swimming yourself if a section of the pool is still open to adults. Go for a long family walk, or meet a mate for a jog and a catch-up, even if it's just for half an hour. Walk the dog that little bit further.

Think about something in your life that you're good at, whether it's work, family life or keeping your home spick and span. Now apply that same discipline, dedication and love to your weight loss, regardless of what day of the week it is. You can achieve anything you want to, whenever you want to.

MY WEIGHT LOSS HAS PLATEAUED. WHAT SHOULD I DO?

Sometimes a diet produces great initial results but then the body grinds to a bit of a halt and decides it's happy with where it is for a while before it's ready to go a step further. Don't worry, your body will take you to the next level eventually, and you'll probably notice a good loss when it does. In the meantime, you need to keep going with the healthy eating and exercise and not lose your momentum. Don't let yourself get bored, as that is fatal on many levels. Boredom means you've lost sight of your goal. Keep things as interesting and varied as you can, and keep the faith. If you're eating less and moving more, you will lose weight!

Also remember that plateauing isn't necessarily a bad thing. It depends where you've got to! If you've slimmed down to a size you're happy with, and your body settles at that weight, then that's amazing. It's what you were aiming for all along! It might not be healthy or necessary for you to lose any more weight, so make sure you're keeping things in perspective.

WHEN IS THE RIGHT TIME TO START A LIFESTYLE OVERHAUL?

Right now! It needn't be seasonal, it's nothing to do with the day of the week, and you don't have to wait until after a massive blowout or a 'final hurrah' to do it. Some people think, 'I'll do it when I get back from holiday – I'll only ruin it all then, anyway.' Their holiday might not be until six months later, but they'll use it as an excuse to carry on eating rubbish.

HOW CAN I SWITCH OFF AND UNWIND?

As well as having long baths, I love listening to the sound of waves on YouTube. I find it's like a Dyson for the mind. It sucks out all the stress or craziness that has built up, especially if I've been learning lines.

If you're working out a lot, your body and your mind will crave relaxation, and you need it. Meditation is incredible for calming down a busy head, and breaks are so important. Or you could do an exercise class that involves choreography, like zumba or step aerobics. These tend to keep your mind so busy thinking about the movements that everything else naturally switches off.

I'M USED TO BEING THE BIG BUBBLY PERSON AND I'M WORRIED I'LL BECOME SHYER IF I LOSE WEIGHT. DID THAT HAPPEN TO YOU?

Definitely not. I'm still me, I'm just a smaller version. Because I no longer drink, I don't tolerate as much crap as I used to, but that's a good thing. Before, I was outwardly confident but my internal self-esteem wasn't great, so that's been a big change. My self-esteem has rocketed since I've lost weight, and so will yours. It didn't happen overnight, but I noticed things gradually shifting. It was wonderful. You'll notice little changes taking place as you go along. It might be that one day you suddenly think to yourself, 'I'm being much less critical of myself these days!' That's when you know this plan is really working for you.

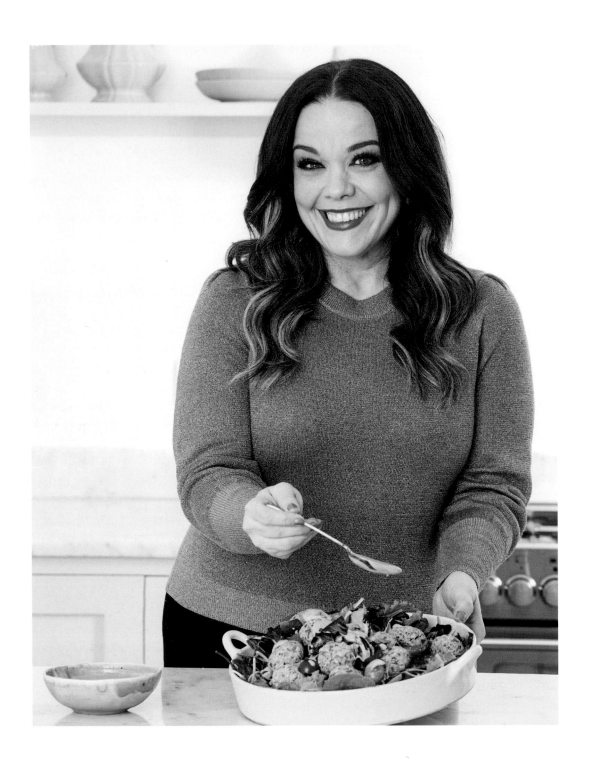

I have days now when I feel like bloody Kylie. I'm more energetic and I'm more positive. I know that an early morning workout is worth the effort, because I'll feel so good once it's done. You really want to get to the point where you look in the mirror and think, 'I'm all right, me.'

DID YOU LOSE WEIGHT FOR OTHER PEOPLE?

Of course I wanted to be healthier so that my loved ones wouldn't worry about me, but ultimately I did it for me. My partner, my friends and my family all loved me the way I was, but I wanted to love myself as much as they did. I did it fully for myself. Fully. You are the only person you can do it for.

I'M WORRIED ABOUT THE REACTION FROM PEOPLE WHEN THEY REALIZE THAT I CAN'T BE THEIR PIZZA OR BURGER BUDDY ANY MORE. HOW DID YOU HANDLE THAT?

I still get stick from people on a daily basis about what I put in my mouth, especially from my family. They'll be eating a four-course Chinese banquet, and while that doesn't bother me a bit, it bothers them that I'm not. They'll call me 'Mini Micro' and ask if I'm having dust for dinner. It's important not to let this kind of thing get you down. I just laugh it off, safe in the knowledge that I've got a healthy and balanced plate in front of me, full of food that I genuinely enjoy eating.

We all went out for a big Christmas lunch last year and there were five courses with different options for each. Everyone else ate all five courses but I only wanted two, so I went for the halibut and scallop options, because honestly, that's all I wanted. I couldn't have physically eaten all that food, but boy, did I get some stick for it! I don't mind what other people eat or how much they weigh. Or whether every single member of my family went home and wolfed down four Chocolate Oranges after the Christmas meal. Do whatever makes you happy, I say. But personally, overeating and then feeling rubbish would not have made me happy. It's as simple as that.

People are also suspicious about what I eat. I get asked over and over again if I'm really as healthy as I say I am. Honestly, if I wasn't I would not look the way I do. I was in the supermarket recently buying all the same foods I always get – avocados, eggs, salad, fish and prawns – and I cannot tell you the number of people who stopped and peered really intently into my basket to see what I was buying. I'm sure they expected me to be hiding a couple of chocolate cakes under a giant bag of lettuce leaves.

My advice would be to be honest with people. Tell them you're doing this for your health and well-being and that you really want to stick with it so you can be happier. Also let them know that it doesn't bother you one bit if they eat pizza in front of you. That should make them feel less guilty (which, let's be honest, is what most food shaming is about).

I SEE RASPBERRY KETONES ADVERTISED ALL OVER SOCIAL MEDIA. HAVE YOU EVER TAKEN THEM?

No, I do not, and I never have. Pictures of me were used without my knowledge or permission as 'the face' of raspberry ketones for a while. After someone let me know about this, I found adverts with my face plastered on them and fake quotes telling everyone how great I thought they were. The truth is that until I got accused of taking them I didn't have a clue what they were – I had to google them! I discovered that a lot of those kinds of tablets contain an ingredient that suppresses hunger, which is not a safe, healthy or sustainable way to lose weight. You're not teaching yourself new habits by taking pills. They're also counterproductive because a lot of them contain ingredients that keep you awake, making you too tired to do any exercise the following day!

As well as being accused of taking pills, I also find it hilarious, not to mention frustrating, that people still think I've had a gastric band fitted, even though I've been very clear and have got concrete proof that I haven't. I get asked about it all the time, as if I'm suddenly going to throw my hands up and say, 'It's a fair cop, you've caught me out. I've been hoodwinking the nation all along.'

I REALLY WORRY ABOUT THE HEALTH IMPLICATIONS OF BEING OVERWEIGHT. HAS LOSING WEIGHT HAD A BIG EFFECT ON YOUR HEALTH?

Absolutely. I'm the healthiest I've ever been. I've had all sorts of tests recently and they've shown I'm in peak condition, and it feels amazing. I no longer have to worry so much about developing type 2 diabetes or other weight-related illnesses or conditions.

I didn't just lose weight when I changed my lifestyle. I also rid myself of a huge amount of worry about my health, and it will be the same for you too. Imagine being able to run around after your kids or sprinting for the bus without getting out of breath. Imagine waking up full of energy ready to face the day. And imagine feeling safe in the knowledge that your body is healthy, inside and out. That's your future.

DO I HAVE TO STOP DRINKING ALCOHOL COMPLETELY ON YOUR PLAN?

Don't hate me, but I would say it's best to in the early days, if you really want to get the results you're after. I'm not saying that everyone has to go teetotal for the rest of their life (though my loved-ones do call me the Booze Gestapo!). But if you want big changes, you're not going to get them as quickly or as easily if you're excessively drinking because it does hamper weight loss. As well as the problem of drunk eating, your body has to burn off alcohol calories before it burns off fat, so putting alcohol into your system does inhibit weight loss. Also, if you're hung-over the last thing you feel like doing is a session in the gym, so it's going to hold you back in that way too.

If you've read my *Honesty Diet* you'll know that drinking used to be a big part of my life. I reckon quite a few people think I still have the odd sneaky tipple behind closed doors. My boyfriend, Al, left half a bottle of red wine in my hotel room when he came to stay recently. When the cleaner saw it she laughed and said, 'You said on *Loose Women* you don't drink, but look!' I must have told her ten times it wasn't mine, but she kept rolling her eyes at me in a 'Yeah, sure!' kind of way and smiling knowingly. I guess I have to accept that there may always be question marks over my lifestyle and that's just how it is.

I often get asked in interviews if I quit booze because I was an alcoholic or had a drink problem. But the simple fact is I was a binge drinker who grew up and came out the other side. Once I'd decided I was done with it, I found I was able to stop straight away, but I know it's not that easy for a lot of people. I actually found smoking much harder to give up, because I based my work life around fag breaks, but everyone has different battles.

If you told me I'd have to experience one of my old hangovers again tomorrow I'd probably cry. They were awful and I don't know how I managed to function when I had one. I didn't ever skip work or let people down due to hangovers, but there were days when it was such a struggle to get through the day. All I could focus on was getting into bed that night.

I no longer have those crazy evenings out where I feel like I'm having the best time because I've drunk so much wine. But I also don't have the crashing lows that would kick in the next morning when I was hung-over, tired, bloated and worrying about what I'd said and done the night before.

Happiness for me now is being able to get up and go to the gym on a Saturday morning and know I've got the whole day ahead of me. Seriously, that is a successful Friday night to me.

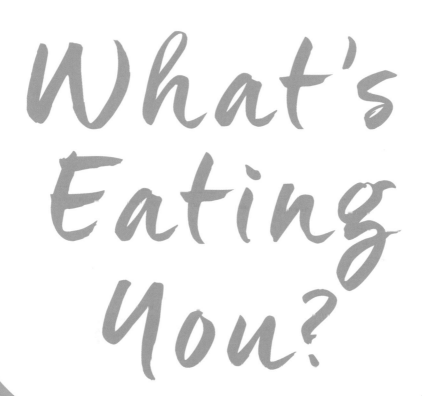

CHAPTER 5

What's Eating You?

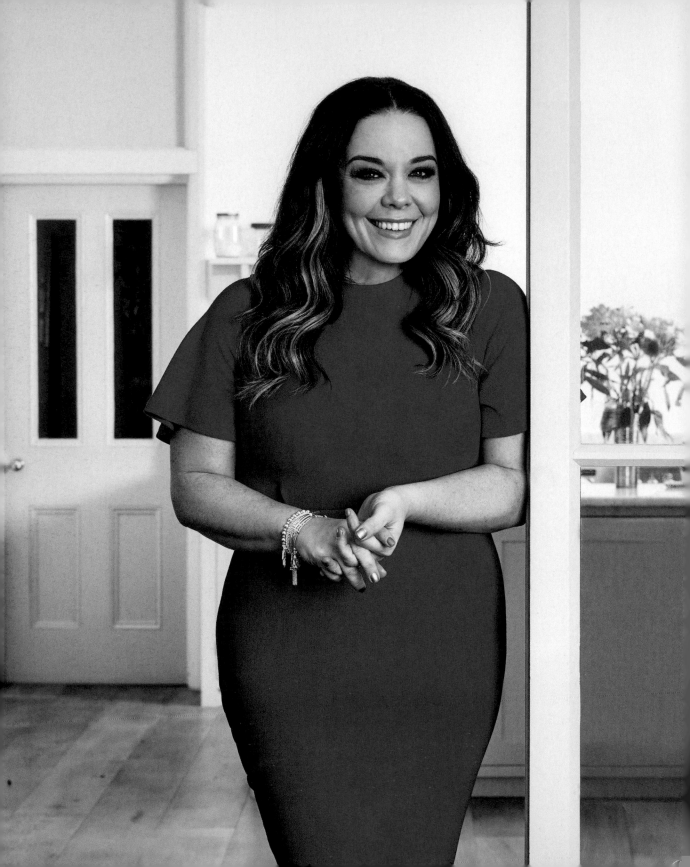

I want to say right now that just because you're going to be eating more healthily, this doesn't mean you can't still adore food and get a huge amount of pleasure from it. I certainly don't feel miserable when I sit down to a nutritious meal – in fact, I feel great about it – and even though I've been eating like this for a few years now, I still find it really exciting discovering new foods and recipes. I'm excited about you doing the same, and you might just surprise yourself when you start branching out and experimenting.

Since I wrote the recipes in my *Honesty Diet*, I've been getting even more adventurous when it comes to food. Beetroot is my new favourite thing, especially combined with pear. I cut two circles of beetroot and put a slice of pear in the middle, and it's utterly delicious. Take my word for it! It's also great with pomegranate, like the recipe on page 224. I love mixing up savoury and sweet these days, and I've also started snacking on popcorn. A handful of salted popcorn is great to tide you over – but that does not mean you can eat the whole bag! Remember: less gets more results.

I adore pulses, whereas I used to avoid them because I didn't know how to cook them. Once you know how to use them to make amazing dishes, you'll be all over them. Preparation is key with my job, and I always thought pulses were annoying and time-consuming. But they're really not, as you'll see from some of the recipes in this book.

LISA'S FOODIE Q&A

Right, now I'm going to answer some of the important food-related questions I often get asked.

IT'S REALLY HARD TO FIND HEALTHY SNACKS WHEN I'M ON THE GO. HOW CAN I AVOID BEING TEMPTED TO GRAB A BAR OF SOMETHING SUGARY?

Healthy food is all around you. You just need to look in the right places. One of my friends said to me recently, 'Why don't places like Starbucks sell fruit so you've got a healthy option when you go there?' Here's the thing: they do! But you only see it if you're looking for it. If you're more interested in cakes and biscuits, the fruit basket probably looks more like decoration than a viable option.

We're also very easily distracted by aromas. As soon as you walk into a coffee shop you'll be hit with the delicious sweetness of freshly baked cakes and the seductive smell of coffee. And let's face it, that doesn't make us fancy a black Americano. I travel by train a lot and when I walk out of a particular station I'm always hit in the face by the smell coming from the Cornish pasty shop. It wakens up your appetite and pulls you in. But believe it or not, they also have nut and seed bags on the counter, so you can go for a healthy treat if you want one.

WHY IS PROTEIN SO GOOD FOR YOU?

As well as keeping you fuller for longer, protein slows down digestion – which makes you less likely to want more food after you've eaten it. It also uses more calories than fat or carbs to process. And it promotes and aids muscle repair, so it's ideal to eat after exercising.

WHY DO PEOPLE ON DIETS HATE CARBS?

Hate is a strong word, but processed carbs like white bread and white rice are not ideal for dieters because they can cause blood-sugar spikes, which ultimately make us feel hungrier again sooner. Good carbs like fruit, vegetables, beans and wholegrains get absorbed more slowly, keeping us fuller for longer, which is why they're a better option by far. And funnily enough, they also contain a lot more nutrients.

Personally, I don't tend to eat carbs after about 2.30 p.m. We naturally lose energy from 3 p.m. onwards, so our bodies don't burn off carbs as quickly. For that reason, I try to have my carbs with my breakfast and my lunch. Your body needs a chance to break them down. But do what is realistic for you, and make any changes like this slowly and sensibly.

When I do eat non-fruit- or non-vegetable-based carbs I'll mainly have oats for breakfast, and quinoa in salads or with fish for lunch. I don't eat any kind of bread and I seriously can't ever see myself eating it again, but that's a personal choice. If you can't bear to give it up completely, switch to a wholemeal variety and try to cut right down so you only have it very occasionally and in tiny amounts. Sandwiches are not essential – your favourite filling can be popped on to a fresh mixed salad instead, or you can use an omelette or lettuce leaves as wraps.

I also don't eat white potatoes, as I find them very easy to overeat and it's far too tempting to load them with butter or cheese. Again, it's my peronal choice, but if you're really intent on losing weight,

I believe it's a choice worth making. If you decide not to cut them out completely, remember that moderation is key.

HOW MUCH FRUIT IS TOO MUCH?

Of course fruit contains sugars, albeit natural ones, but I love it. Grapes and little scoops or cubes of kiwi fruit are great for tickling your palate. The sharper the better, in my opinion. Berries are good too. I tend to go for the darker ones because I prefer the taste, so I eat a lot of blueberries, raspberries and cranberries. And if I am making a smoothie I'll mix fruit with vegetables and a good squirt of lime juice. Having three fruit-based smoothies a day would be way, way too much sugar, and I certainly don't eat fruit all day every day, but it is still a great snack.

WHY DO YOU RECOMMEND EATING DINNER EARLY?

I don't eat after 6.30 p.m. so that I give my body time to have a complete rest and a chance to break down the day's food before I go to bed. It's been one of my main rules for a long time now, and I only break it if something major gets in the way – for instance, if I have to work late and there are no healthy food options available at the right time.

I always make lunch my main meal so that my body has the whole afternoon to process it. If you're eating enough for breakfast, lunch and dinner, even if you stop eating at 6.30 p.m. you shouldn't feel the need for late-night snacks.

I know it's tricky if you work nine to five, or if you've got to collect kids from after-school clubs, but if this is the case make sure you have some pre-prepared food ready for when you get home. Take a look at the 'Get Ahead' section of the recipes (see page 191) and batch cook in advance so you have something waiting in your kitchen that's ready to eat in minutes.

WHAT'S SO GREAT ABOUT WATER?

We're told every day how great water is for our body and our skin, but it's also the dieter's friend. It's easy to mistake thirst for hunger, so if you're feeling peckish, first have a pint of water with a squeeze of lemon or lime juice, or a herbal tea. Give yourself twenty minutes to work out if you really do need a snack or if the water has done the job.

WHEN SHOULD I DO MY BIG SUPERMARKET SHOP?

Never when you're hungry! You will end up buying things you don't need. Deliveries are so much safer because you only put what you planned to buy in your online basket. We've talked about the dangers and temptations you will face in the supermarket. I know people who eat on the way around the shop and then pay for it at the end because the impulse to snack is just too much. Get too grabby and you'll soon get flabby!

I'M GOING ON HOLIDAY. DO I HAVE TO PUT MY DIET ON HOLD?

This question drives me a bit mad. You do not have to overfeed yourself on holiday. It's not compulsory. You can eat really well and swim every day or go for long walks. Your healthy lifestyle does not have to go out of the window just because you're in another country. Letting go on holiday does not have to include your eating habits. If you're in a hotel, embrace the salad bar. If you're in a self-catered apartment, buy fresh local food. And avoid pina coladas!

I've seen the most incredible gluttony on cruises, to the point where I didn't understand how people could fit that much food in. And remember in the old days I could really pack it away, so that's saying something!

You need these ingredients to stay healthy: dedication, motivation and willpower. Once you master them, you're set for life. Eating healthily will become second nature, whether you're on holiday or not.

I ALWAYS WANT TO SNACK WHEN I'M SITTING IN FRONT OF THE TV AT NIGHT. WHAT SHOULD I DO?

Advertisers put all the food ads on at night, so you're vulnerable while you're watching TV. It's no wonder you're tempted! You're a captive audience, and evenings are prime snacking time, so watch yourself. The best thing you can do is record the programme and watch it on a delay, so you can whizz through the ads. If you've had enough food for lunch and dinner, you shouldn't want to snack. But if you are really desperate, snack on some fruit or a few protein-packed nuts, though ideally not too close to bedtime. Or have a cup of herbal tea to check it's not thirst you're feeling.

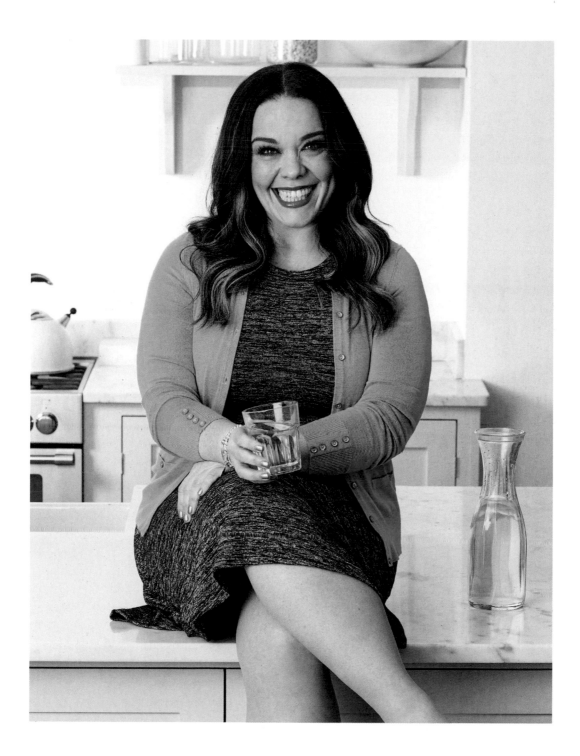

WHAT DO I DO IF I HAVE TO EAT A SET MEAL AT A WEDDING OR A PARTY?

See the good on the plate and just eat the healthy stuff. No one says you must eat everything. And you can ask for less food. The mouth you eat with can also speak, and the world isn't going to crumble if you ask to have your meal with extra vegetables instead of chips. If there's a choice of meals, you could always pre-order the vegan or vegetarian option, which is often healthier – though check what it is first, don't just assume it will be!

WHAT DO I DO IF I'M GOING TO A PARTY WHERE THERE WILL BE LOADS OF TEMPTING FOODS?

Eat a meal beforehand so you're not tempted to pick. If it's a buffet or canapés, no one is going to notice whether you're eating or not.

I NEVER FEEL HUNGRY IN THE MORNING AND I OFTEN MAKE DO WITH JUST A COFFEE. IS THAT BAD?

Yes! Breakfast is so important for fuelling your body for the rest of the day. Your energy levels will suffer if you don't put in the right things. If you absolutely have to miss your evening meal that's bad enough, but even that is preferable to missing breakfast. You need to keep stoking the nutritional fire.

THERE'S LOTS OF UNHEALTHY FOOD IN MY HOUSE FOR MY PARTNER OR KIDS. HOW CAN I RESIST THE TEMPTATION?

Have your own cupboard where you keep your own foods, and avoid looking in the other ones as much as possible. Of course it's hard if you have to cook for the family and give the kids their treats. But other than that, avoid them. Get your other half to hide the naughty stuff so you don't know where it is. And this may sound mad, but even if you don't have kids, put child locks on all the cupboards apart from your own healthy one so you have to think twice before you open them. In that moment when you go to open the cupboard door and 'just have one biscuit' you will have a chance to stop yourself.

Put Post-it notes on your cupboard with messages telling yourself how well you're doing or stick up your worst photos to remind you how you *don't* want to look. Find the humour in dieting. If you go five days without any sugar, stick up a Post-it note reminding yourself of that. We congratulate kids when they do well, so why not ourselves? You could even go a step further and get stickers to put in your Honesty Diary and give yourself one, two or three stars depending on how well you've done. Bring the fun back to it!

WHERE TO EAT OUT

I travel a lot for work so, wherever I am, if I'm eating out I scour the local area for places to eat and make sure to choose restaurants that serve things that are healthy and suit my eating plan. I don't take a chance on going to a restaurant only to discover that they specialize in burgers and chips and offer no alternatives. I check menus online and I plan ahead.

When I was working in Manchester last year filming the BBC drama *Age Before Beauty* I had to live in a hotel for over four months. Before I got there, I looked at the hotel's room-service menu and there was only one thing on it (a spinach, sun-dried tomato and pine nut salad) that I felt I could eat. The rest of it was full-on junk food. If you ever find yourself in a situation like this, where it seems like work or life is throwing obstacles at you and your diet, my advice is not to panic. You just need to stop, think and take action. In this instance, I found a nearby supermarket and every day after filming I would go and buy a packet of salmon and some interesting salads, or something similar. I deliberately made good choices so I didn't end up with any 'Sod it, I'll grab something from Greggs' instances. I would have my big meal at lunchtime, on location, where they served healthier options, such as fish and vegetables, and when I got back to the hotel each night I made sure my evening meal was to hand so I wasn't tempted to order a pizza.

I am very aware of how easy it can be to fall off the food wagon and go back to old ways. Over time, I've become super vigilant about this, so that I don't slip back into eating countless pieces of white toast with rivers of butter running through them. I refuse to let my old habits come creeping back!

I'm not perfect, and of course I am tempted to indulge sometimes – mainly when it's my time of the month. But I generally find the strength not to, because I know it's a bad road for me to go down.

None of us are perfect. It's all about finding that place where we feel happiest, and working out what suits us and keeps us on track. For me, that's being pretty strict most of the time, but for someone else it may mean staying on track six days a week so they can enjoy a little treat on a Sunday.

I was never that girl who was a couple of sizes larger than average and just wanted to lose a few pounds. I was obese! To this day I have to throw everything I've got at my weight loss and at maintaining my healthier diet and body shape. And that's why I make sure I'm always prepared.

I'm all about the planning, so if you find yourself needing to buy food when you're travelling or eating out, these are your best options at each of the main high-street restaurants and food retailers.

PRET A MANGER
The healthy Pret pots and soups are great, and they've got a really wide selection. But sorry, no bread with your soup!

CAFÉ ROUGE
They do some lovely salads (but watch out for those creamy dressings). Or you could go for chicken or steak with vegetables, but hold the garlic butter.

PREZZO
The sea bass is a brilliant choice, and the goat's cheese and beetroot salad is a winner, but I'm afraid you'll have to park the garlic bread.

NANDO'S
Again, Nando's offer some good salads, but beware of creamy dressings. A plain chicken breast is great. You can have a bit of sauce on the side, and enjoy with corn on the cob or chargrilled vegetables.

MCDONALD'S
Surprisingly McDonald's sell porridge for a morning post-gym pick-me-up, as well as carrot sticks, fruit bags and a healthy chicken salad.

MARKS & SPENCER
I adore both the sun-dried tomato and the salmon salads. Of course you can also pick up loads of fruits, veg and salads, and easy-to-nibble packets of cooked prawns or chicken pieces. The same goes for other supermarkets.

PIZZA EXPRESS

Pizza Express is another great place for salads, especially the Leggera Superfood option, but again shoo away the dough sticks. You could also have olives to start, and a raspberry sorbet for dessert if you really need something sweet.

CHINESE

Chinese is tricky, because it can be loaded with salt and saturated fats. But king prawn and pineapple (ask for it as plain as possible), stir-fried vegetables and any clear soups are all top of the healthy list.

INDIAN

Much like Chinese, Indian food can have a lot of sneaky hidden fats – even the vegetables! Chicken or prawn tandoori dishes are preferable, because they're cooked in a clay oven without sauces, but sadly naan breads are out.

THAI

Tom yum soup is absolutely delicious and diet friendly, as are plain stir-fries, grilled fish or chicken satay (but ask for the sauce on the side and only have a little). Papaya salad often contains quite a lot of sugar but it's still one of the best things on the menu.

KFC

Pretty much everything in KFC is fried, but the best of a bad bunch is the Original Recipe Salad.

BURGER KING

Yet more fast food! But if you're desperate I would recommend the Crispy Chicken Salad. Add the Apple Fries from the kids' menu (they're basically chopped apple but they're a good sweet hit).

GOURMET BURGER KITCHEN

Go for any kind of burger without the bun, served with a large salad (dressing on the side!).

TURKISH

There are lots of great things on offer at Turkish restaurants. Meat, fish and chicken shish kebabs skewered with vegetables are packed with protein and nutrients, and fresh olives and crisp salads are perfect accompaniments.

GREEK

One of my favourite things to eat in Greek restaurants is grilled halloumi. But small is beautiful so it's best to share a portion with someone. Grilled skewers of meat are also readily available, as are cold meat platters and delicious veggies.

MEXICAN

Mexican restaurants are so delicious, but so dangerous! A good tip is to ask for no taco shells but plenty of lettuce with your meal so you can make lettuce wraps filled with grilled fish, chicken or vegetables.

WAGAMAMA

Wagamama is a funny one because some of the healthier-looking dishes aren't actually the best choices. Edamame beans and miso soup are great starters, and for a main course the ramen soups are a safe bet, as are the wok-fried greens and grilled tuna.

JAPANESE

I can eat sushi until the cows come home and I would always recommend it to people (if you're a raw fish fan, that is), but try not to have too many of the white-rice-based offerings. Stick to the raw fish dishes and feel free to go to town on the miso soup.

GREGGS

Believe it or not, you can find healthy options in Greggs these days. They've moved on from just mayo-laden sandwiches and pies and they now offer soups and salads, as well as fruit.

PIZZA HUT

Thanks to the unlimited salad buffet it is possible to eat well in a Pizza Hut, but go easy on the heavy dressings. And if you fancy something sweet, the mango sorbet is refreshing and (almost) guilt free.

FISH AND CHIPS

Oh, come on . . .

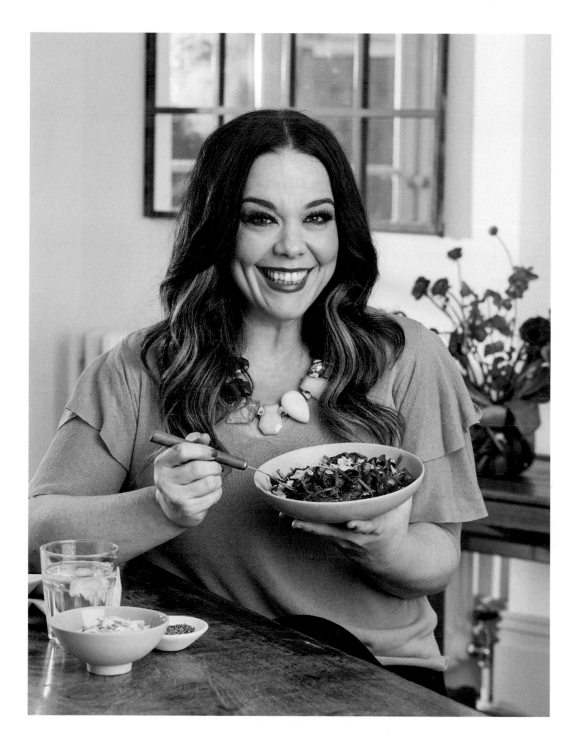

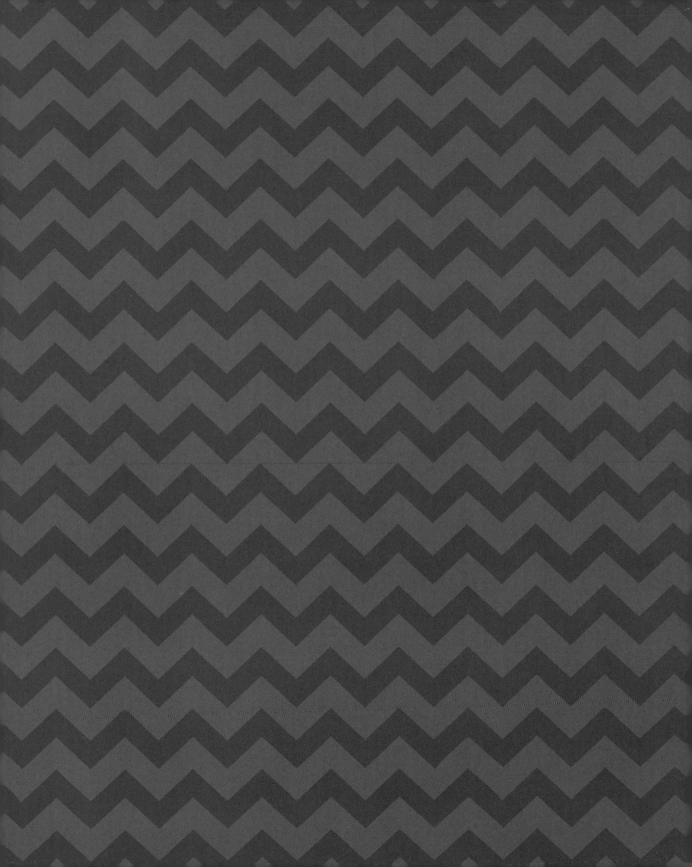

CHAPTER 6

Movers and Shakers

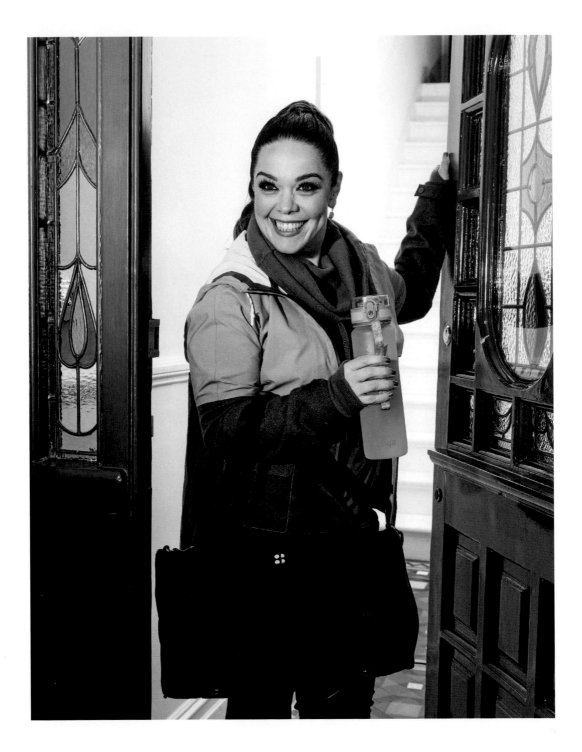

This may be the section you're tempted to skip through because you think eating well is enough to make you lose weight. Bad news, everyone! Diet and exercise go hand in hand. They're like spaghetti and Bolognese.

When people are young they can go on a diet and drop half a stone in two weeks and they will look the same, only smaller, because their body retains its shape. Maybe if I'd gone on a massive diet in my twenties, when my skin was tighter, I wouldn't have needed my skin-removal operations because my body would have snapped back into shape. Who knows?

But if you're older, or you've got a serious amount of weight to lose, you are going to need to work out in order to tone up. As we age, our body doesn't ping back as easily. So you need to help it get into its new shape. Find your groove, then your move!

It feels like a lot has changed since I wrote my *Honesty Diet* in terms of new workouts I've discovered and new foods I've fallen in love with. I'm eating things I once never imagined I would, and my diet is a million miles away from the giant bags of crisps and supersized bars of chocolate I used to fill my trolley with.

I've upped my exercise levels even more and I sometimes work out six days a week, which I know sounds like a crazy amount, especially if you're just starting out. (Don't worry, you don't need to do as much as me to see a difference – every little bit of exercise helps!) I love exercise so much now that I even hired a spin bike for my hotel room when I was doing panto in Wolverhampton last winter. While the rest of the cast went out drinking after the shows, Nana here would head back to her room to shower and go to bed so she could get up early to squeeze in some exercise. The show, *Jack and the Beanstalk,* was a great form of cardio in itself too. I was moving around on stage non-stop, especially during some of the more energetic skits, and we were doing two shows a day so I was constantly moving my body. I felt super fit and very happy to have a job that involved so much built in activity!

Nowadays I still work out with a personal trainer, and on top of that I'll often do half an hour on my own, either in the gym, at home, or in a hotel room if I'm away working. I plan out everything I do to make sure there's a way for me to fit in or incorporate exercise. I fully realize that not everyone can afford a personal trainer or an exercise bike in their hotel room (that was a massive luxury for me), but I'll also find zumba or aerobics routines online and do them in front of my laptop or the TV. There are so many apps and pay-as-you-go gyms too. There is no excuse for me to slack off.

I find it so much easier to exercise these days, but it wasn't an overnight thing. As I said in my last book, I didn't become a gym bunny in a matter of days. I started off slowly by doing aqua aerobics classes when I was at my biggest, and I gradually built things up to where I am today. I am testament to the fact that if you stick at something you can achieve whatever you want to. I've trained my brain and body to get into that zone, and it's taken work.

Am I strict with myself now? Yes, but I'm honest about that. Some people live on steamed vegetables but pretend they go out for lavish dinners every night. I'm not one of those people, and I never will be. I'm realistic about what I put in my mouth, and I always tell the truth about it.

GETTING THE BOOT

I'm always up for trying new things when it comes to exercise and I love pushing myself, and it's for that reason I ended up doing an intensive week-long boot camp last year. Me being me, I didn't go in soft and try out an easy one first. I went to one of the more advanced ones you can do, and it was a real challenge. As you know, I'm used to exercising now and I do love it, but this was constant. We were up at 5 a.m. going for a ramble, and we didn't stop exercising for the rest of the day. We were doing classes, running, squatting – you name it.

For breakfast we'd have one poached egg and one piece of smoked salmon, for lunch we'd have an onion and broccoli omelette with some rocket, and for dinner we'd have cauliflower soup or a vegetable broth. We'd have protein balls made with dates, peanut butter and coconut for a morning snack, and a hard-boiled egg for an afternoon snack. It was less food than I usually eat. I remember being given three sticks of celery and some chilli hummus as a snack one afternoon and I thought Christmas had come early!

Challenging as it was, it took my training to another level and the results were mind-blowing. I don't mean in terms of how much I weighed, because I make a point of not jumping on the scales every five minutes, but in terms of how different my body felt. By the end of the camp I'd lost five inches from around my upper body, five inches around my waist and four on my hips and bum. The only place I didn't lose any weight was my arms, which is surprising because I was doing so much boxing, as well as one-armed press-ups and burpees.

Our trainer, Danny, was an ex-marine and he pushed us hard but I loved him to death. There's nothing I like more than someone giving me a good kick up the backside and spurring me on. At one point Danny said to me, 'Blimey, you've got legs like Serena Williams,' and I thought,

'That'll do me fine!' Because I'm little, they're like rocks now and very toned, and that's what I always wanted. I love that athletic look. I was ready for a break by the end of the week, but also on a real high. And yes, I would do it again!

I know this sounds full-on, and it was, and you probably think I'm mad. But I'm telling you this story as an example of what can be achieved in the long term. I would never expect you to sign up to a week of intensive exercise, but when you consider that a few years ago I could barely walk to the bus stop without complaining, it just shows what a change of mindset and dedication can do. And whether you realize it or not yet, you've got that inside of you, however you choose to find it.

I also met some amazing people on the boot camp, and we all motivated each other so much. That week taught me not just to go the extra mile, but to go the extra few miles. I cannot tell you how well I slept there. It was incredible. And each day I woke up ready to take on another session (well, most mornings!).

I'm still in touch with lots of those people now. That's been another massively positive side effect of having a new lifestyle. I've met so many new people, and they're not just interested in me because of my job. We've got a common interest and loads to talk about, and I adore that. I met one woman who has a really similar body shape to me now, and she used to be a size 20. I'm so proud of her. Seeing other people achieve their goals inspires me so much because it also highlights how much I've changed.

Another example is Lisa, forty-three, who I met while promoting my previous book. She says:

'I'd tried every diet going, but I needed some solid, realistic guidance, and Lisa gave me that. My main goals were to change my eating patterns and feel better about myself, and I've done both of those things and more. I had a rough year in 2017 and put on a lot of weight, but I'm now eating much more healthily, I've broken bad habits, I've got more control over what I'm putting in my mouth and I feel more positive.

My two kids are also eating better. They can see that I'm making better choices so they are too. I'm cooking them meals from Lisa's book and we're all trying new things. I had no idea I liked avocado so much!

These days, I take my dog out for a long walk every day, and I've joined a gym and go at least three times a week. I go with my daughter or my parents so it's a real family affair. I've started to really enjoy it, which I never thought I would say. I can see changes in my body already and I feel like I'm in a different place. Taking that first step changed everything.'

DO WHAT WORKS FOR YOU

Step tabata is a new exercise workout I've discovered, which is a form of high-intensity interval training (HIIT) that's broken up into four-minute sessions. It's not for the faint-hearted but it feels so good. And I've also been trying out a new ski dancing workout which is so much fun. You really feel it the following day because you're constantly in a squat position while you're working out. But you just know it's lifting your bum right up where it should be.

One class I love more than any other I've tried in a long time is 'Back to the 80s', where you work out with glow sticks. I get to do old-school aerobics to all my old favourite Hacienda dance tunes. How cool is that? It's like the eighties never ended, and I have such a brilliant time that the classes fly by. I did my classes in Manchester but they're starting up all over the country, so have a look online and see if there are any near you.

I love the fact that old-fashioned aerobics is coming back into fashion. It worked back in the eighties so why would it not still work today? It's only a matter of time before I'm wearing bright pink Lycra and a sweatband! Classes do follow trends, and there's always something new coming out, so you need to decide what works for you and not do it just because it's 'trendy'. If you want to buy into a new fad, why not? You might love it. But don't feel you have to try something just because all the magazines are telling you to.

On a very simplistic level I've been doing more walking than ever, which I absolutely love. It's a part of my regime these days. I would always rather walk somewhere than get a bus or a taxi. Obviously I'm not about to start walking from London to Manchester any time soon. But if it's a short journey that I can power-walk, I'm all over it. If the journey is that bit too far, I'll cycle. I am so in love with cycle hire schemes – they're easy, cheap and cycling really gets your heart going.

TO GYM OR NOT TO GYM?

I'm more than aware that the gym is not for everyone. Some people love it, others not so much. I do belong to a gym, but mainly because it's just around the corner from my house and as I'm so short on time it's a handy way to fit in my exercise. But I'd be just as happy with a local sports centre. You don't need to go to a pricey boot camp or a fancy gym to get into shape. When I was away working in another city recently, I would go along to the local church hall and work out with a load of local ladies. It was so much fun! And as you'll see from the workouts later in this book (see pages 102–21), the chances are you've got everything you need at home.

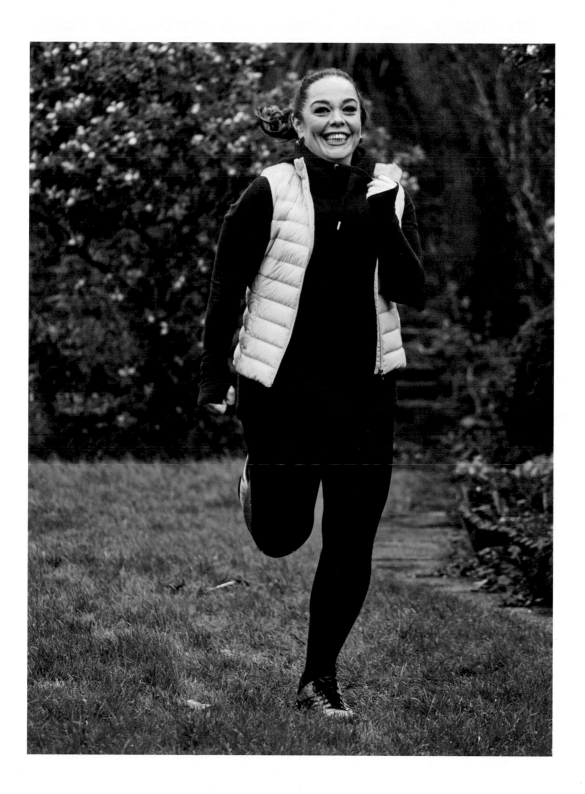

FIND YOUR EXERCISE TRIBE

Try different gyms, leisure centres or classes and find where you feel comfortable. If you were buying a house you wouldn't snap up the very first one you looked round. You would do extensive research and find the one that's right for you. It's the same with exercise. This is somewhere where you're (ideally!) going to spend a lot of time, so it's important for you to find one that suits you. Don't be scared to go back for a second viewing, either. If you can't decide, you could try Pay As U Gym, which gives you access to loads of different places, so you can mix and match depending on your mood.

ASK FOR ADVICE

If you haven't ever stepped into a gym before, or not for many years, don't be embarrassed to ask for help. Please don't bowl in there and start using the machines without asking for advice. It's what the gym instructors are there for. Don't just stick a pin in any hold on the bench press and hope for the best. You really need to know what you're doing or you could end up injuring yourself.

If you're using free weights you can't go straight from 4kg to 10kg because you happen to be feeling strong that day. You could end up counteracting exactly what you're trying to do. You're not a bodybuilder, and you're not looking to have Arnie arms. Certain weights will tone and lengthen your muscles while others will simply bulk you up, and you always want the former. You will be just as strong, but you will be in the shape you want to be in – unless, of course, you want to look like Arnie!

I would also recommend trying a kettle bells class before you start doing weights, to see if you like it or not. (Kettle bells are ball-shaped weights with a handle on the top, and they can help you reach different muscles to the ones you use with dumb-bells. Flip to page 119 to see what one looks like.) Doing a class is a great way to try them out, plus you can ask the instructor for some advice. I have learned so much about working out now, but I still need advice and help to move forward to the next level.

KEEP THINGS INSPIRING AND INTERESTING

Your body can quickly get used to what it's doing and settle into a routine, so ideally you need to mix things up as often as you can. Once you've done a couple of months of Zumba, switch to something else, perhaps a spin class or find a different Zumba instructor who has new routines and music. Keep your workouts varied, otherwise your body will get used to using the same muscles. You want to keep challenging it by making it do different things. On a very basic level, it keeps things more interesting for you too!

FIND YOUR PACE

When it comes to exercise some people like to drive at 30 mph and some people like to drive at 70. Personally, I'm a 50. Sometimes I speed up and go a bit faster, and sometimes I might go at 40 because I have slightly less energy one day. And what if you need to put the brakes on every now and again and have a little rest? So be it. You can turn on the ignition and start the car up again anytime (I love a good driving analogy).

If you want to start really slowly, that's perfectly fine. Yoga and Pilates do count as exercise if you do them properly. If you just lie on the floor doing some deep breathing and tickling your toe on the ground you are effectively meditating, not exercising. But if you put some effort in you will soon see the toning benefits, and they are a good place to start your exercise journey. Don't feel intimidated by yoga – it's not all handstands! Plank is a yoga pose, don't forget.

ONCE YOU'RE ON A ROLL, PUSH YOURSELF

Once you've got your fitness levels up, I want you to go for it! When you're in the zone, envisage yourself as a candle and watch the fat melt away. Always remember my mantra:

SWEAT IS FAT CRYING!

As well as losing inches on our thighs or waist we want to shed visceral fat, which is internal fatty tissue that clings to our organs. It's a huge reason why people get fatty liver or heart disease, so losing weight is not the only benefit of improved fitness.

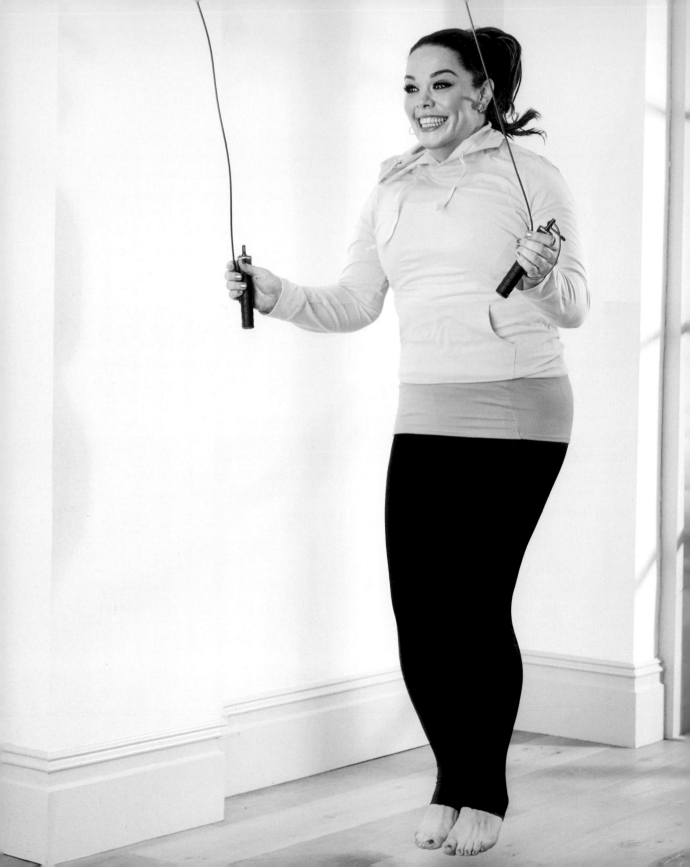

BUT DON'T OVERDO THINGS

I try to put everything into my workouts, but I do give myself a break if I need it. The scar on my left arm (a reminder of my skin-removal surgery) is still quite painful, and during one session I overdid it and had to skip training for a couple of days. My arm felt like someone was holding a lighter underneath it and burning my flesh, which was no fun. That taught me a valuable, if painful, lesson.

There is no mad rush. You're getting yourself into shape for life. Yes, you want to work hard, but you don't want to injure yourself. I don't mind a bit of aching the day after exercising, because that shows I've been working hard – and I like to think it's my body giving me a clap and saying, 'Well done, you gave it your all!' – but I do not like being in genuine pain. The absolute worst thing is pushing your body past its limits and then not being able to exercise for a week. Don't be that person who puts her back out in yoga and then sits around feeling miserable for days on end because she's ruled herself out of classes or can't physically manage a jog around the block.

You want to push yourself just enough so you can achieve what you want, but not so that you injure yourself. Listen to your body. It will tell you when it's had enough. You will soon get to know your body so well, you will know how far you can go with it.

EXERCISE FOR FREE

If you don't like the idea of a gym, I've included lots of home workouts in this book (see pages 102–21), plus there are loads of YouTube videos you can do at home. Or why not start a running group with your mates? Or a speed-walking group, if you don't feel ready to run yet? At least you're getting out and about, and you can finish with some stretching exercises. If you've got friends with kids in prams, do a pacey push. If you're single, grab some local friends and walk and talk. Instead of sitting on the sofa talking to each other on the phone, stick your trainers on and get a good pace going. Talk about your week and offload on each other. Imagine how good you'll feel after a good session of that. You'll be lightening your load and your body at the same time. Loads of parks have free workout equipment in them now. It's become the norm to pop along in your joggers and do some squats, so no one is going to look at you like you're mad.

GET A WORKOUT PAL

Personally, I like working out alone. But if you like company while you're exercising, do it with a friend. You can be each other's personal trainer and push each other to do more. Even if you're screaming at each other and your mate says they hate you, you'll thank each other for it in the long run! You want friends on your side who are going to be cheerleaders, so choose someone you know will have your back as well as their own.

REMEMBER, THIS IS YOUR JOURNEY

Whatever you do when you're working out, please don't look at the woman next to you in Zumba and wonder why you don't have her long legs. It will not help. The only person you should be comparing yourself to when you're exercising is the old you. It's your journey. There's nothing wrong with being motivated by someone else who has got to where you want to be, but don't evaluate yourself based on how someone else looks. For all you know, that person could be jealous of something about you. We all have our strengths. Play to them. Don't think that because someone is slimmer than you they're better. Skinny doesn't mean fit. There are a lot of women who are very slim, but they may not be healthy or strong. There's the whole 'skinny fat' thing, where women can be very slender but also have a fair amount of internal fat. So you could be a lot healthier than them, even if you are a few sizes bigger.

Do you want to stand at the back of a class where no one can see you? Do it. Do you want to stand at the front and give it your all? Get up there. Do whatever makes you comfortable. Stop rolling your eyes at the 'Captain Keenos' who stand right in front of the instructor. If someone wants to be centre stage in a combat class, let them. (Or join them!) Embrace the fact that it's what works for them. Maybe they're short-sighted and can't see the instructor from the back of the hall! Equally, if you want to get to a class twenty minutes early so you can secure a spot in the corner at the back, because you're not feeling confident, what's the problem? At least you're there. No one is right or wrong. Front, middle or back, it makes no odds. You just need to find your place.

The people who get the most out of classes, or in the gym, are the ones who don't care what anyone else is doing because they're totally in their own zone. Wear what you want and do it at your pace. An old T-shirt and leggings are fine. You don't need to be wearing a designer neon kit to do a good workout.

Take it from me, when the penny drops and you realize that your exercise journey is about you and no one else, it's a huge relief.

MAKE WORKOUT TIME FAMILY TIME

A woman stopped me in the street a while ago and said, 'Do you really go for long walks on a Sunday? Why don't you give yourself a break?' The answer is, I don't want one! I love going for long walks with Al to clear out the cobwebs, and then getting home and cosying up for the rest of the day. Sundays seem to last forever. I can have a nice sit down and watch a film later, and I don't feel guilty because I've already been out and about. If you've got kids, bung their coats on and head off for an hour. Do a treasure hunt in the local park or woods and even get some buddies together and do it with their kids too. How much fun is that? Get your whole family involved.

Why not make obstacle courses or enjoy races with your kids in the park? Or have your own sports day? Get prizes for the winners, and you can have a nice (healthy) picnic too. The whole family can get involved and you can all push each other on. Why not buy yourself a spinning light for your front room and have a disco with the kids? Dance until you're completely breathless and there's your workout, right there! And you'll all love it, so you won't even realize you're exercising. Get the kids' feedback about what else they would like to do. They've got never-ending energy, so they'll spur you on.

SPEED UP YOUR EVERYDAY LIFE

It feels like everything in the world is getting faster but we're getting slower and more inactive. We can order our shopping online in ten minutes and get it delivered, so we're not walking to the shops and then carrying our bags home any more. We can download a book or an album in seconds, so we don't have to leave the house to go to the library to get one. Those things are wonderful and helpful in lots of ways, but they're making us lazy. We need to go old-school again. Back in the day, we would go and hire a video from a shop as a family and then sit down and watch it (after spending at least an hour arguing over what we were going to watch, obviously). Once it was over, we'd go and do something else.

These days everything we want to watch is there at the click of a button. Instead of spending two hours stretched out on the sofa watching a movie, we're spending eight hours watching a box set, probably only moving to go to the loo or get food. We're so much more sedentary, so we need to start doing simple, small things that make a big difference. Get up early and go for a jog before you watch that series. Or break the episodes up by going for a walk or running up and down your stairs in the middle. I know from experience how easy it is to spend the entire weekend on the sofa barely moving, and it is not healthy.

Another tip that is so easy and obvious is to walk the kids to school one day instead of taking the car. Just wake up earlier and you can do it. These things don't have to be grand gestures, but small things equal a smaller waist. I run up and down stairs all the time now. And I don't even notice it, because it's second nature. I've programmed myself like a machine.

NO MORE CBB

'Can't be bothered' is not a phrase that should exist in your vocabulary any more. That is now being replaced with 'can be bothered'. If you wake up and it's cold and rainy outside and you don't want to work out, keep repeating 'I can be bothered' and give yourself that kick up the backside you need. Think about what you'll get out of it. If you're feeling down, that run or class will be your saviour. The mental-health benefits of exercise are truly incredible. That's a big part of what drives me to get out of bed and exercise every morning.

START A WORKOUT TIMETABLE

If you've got kids, the chances are they've got a homework timetable, so why not create one for your workouts? At my school we had to get our parents to sign off our homework diaries each day, so you could always get one of your nearest and dearest to check it for you so you know you've stuck to it. Pride yourself on the exercise sessions you've done each week!

Print off a copy of the calendar on your computer, put it up on your fridge and write down all the times you want to do exercise. If you're planning to go to a class on a Monday, don't think, 'Ah, but Cheryl might want to come round that night.' No, she can come round another time.

People get themselves up for work each day, or they get their kids to school, because they must. Treat exercise in the same way. It cannot be the first thing to go if life gets busy. Once it's in the diary, it's scheduled. If you can, pay for classes upfront so you've made a commitment. If you do cancel, write down the reason why on that sheet and you'll soon see a pattern emerge. If it's something you think you need to explore further, write it down in your Honesty Diary and try to work out what's blocking you.

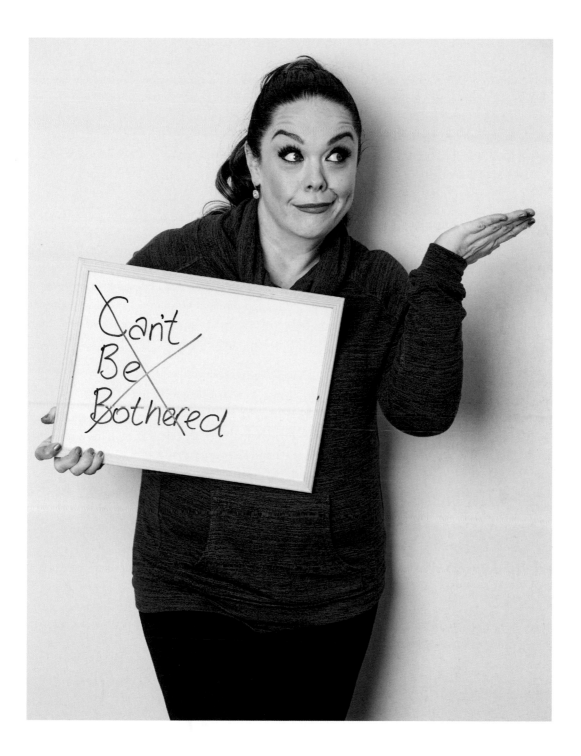

EAT WHEN IT SUITS YOU

Some people eat before their morning workout session and some people don't. Personally, it works for me to eat afterwards, but it's down to you. You know your body, or you will certainly start to, and if you need some porridge to get your body going and give you the oomph to get to the gym, you do that. But whatever you do, do not reward yourself with naughty treats after a workout, or run to the café for a breakfast muffin, because you're so hungry. If you're worried you'll need to eat post-workout, take a healthy snack to the gym with you.

DON'T CLOCK-WATCH

What gets me through when I'm working out is listening to different songs, and that's how I time myself too. I'll ramp up a Five Star song and I'll know when it finishes that I've done about three minutes of exercise. And then it's on to the next song, and the next three minutes. Make yourself some brilliant playlists and the time will fly by. My current favourite selection is opposite.

LET'S GET TO IT!

Okay, we've talked a lot about exercise and now it's time to get down and actually do some. I've created a series of simple workouts that you can do at home, in the local park, or in the gym – the choice is yours. Each workout is laid out on a single page so that you can take a photo of them with your phone, then you've always got them to hand. There really is no excuse!

Each workout is designed to get your heart rate up and your body burning fat, and I've even included a TV workout so you can tone up while you're watching *Corrie*. I'm good like that.

For all the workouts, the aim is to try and achieve as many reps of each exercise as possible in 30 seconds, with a 30–60 second rest between each set.

For all the workouts, try to do 2–3 sets of exercises to begin with, and as you get fitter decrease the rest time in between exercises and add more sets.

Don't forget to warm up and stretch before you start. Off you go!

MY WORKOUT PLAYLIST

'Virtual Insanity' – *Jamiroquai*

'Get Right' – *Jennifer Lopez*

'I See You Baby' – *Groove Armada*

'Cheerleader' – *Omi*

'Wanna Be Startin' Somethin''
– *Michael Jackson*

'Love On Top' – *Beyoncé*

'Domino' – *Jessie J*

'Sign Your Name' – *Terence Trent D'Arby*

'So Good To Me' – *Chris Malinchak*

'Treasure' – *Bruno Mars*

'The Club Is Alive' – *JLS*

'Sing Hallelujah' – *Dr Alban*

'Playing With Knives' – *Bizarre Inc*

'Love Come Down' – *Evelyn 'Champagne' King*

'And The Beat Goes On'
– *The Whispers*

'On And On' – *Erykah Badu*

'Shake Your Body' – *The Jacksons*

'Sweet Harmony' – *The Beloved*

'Too Blind To See It' – *Kym Sims*

'Hold On' – *En Vogue*

'Shake Your Groove Thing'
– *Peaches & Herb*

'Things That Make You Go Hmm...'
– *C+C Music Factory*

'Rhythm Of The Night' – *DeBarge*

'Never Gonna Give You Up'
– *Rick Astley*

'Footloose' – *Kenny Loggins*

'Black Magic' – *Little Mix*

'Feels' – *Calvin Harris*

'Cherish' – *Madonna*

'This Is What You Came For'
– *Calvin Harris*

'Closer' – *Ne-Yo*

THE JUST-MAKE-A-START WORKOUT

Don't know where to start when it comes to exercising? This workout will ease you in perfectly.

1. March on the spot and raise each knee above your waist alternately to increase your heart rate.

2. Sit down on a chair using a squatting motion and stand up again quickly, without using your arms to help. Keep your head and chest up, your lower back tucked in and hold in your stomach.

3. Lie on the floor with your legs bent, your knees together and your arms stretched out above your head holding a cushion. Sit up and reach over your knees to touch your feet with the cushion. Lie back down, placing your arms above your head again. When you improve, stop using the cushion.

4. Go down on to your hands and knees and keep your head raised so you're looking out in front of you. Hold one arm out straight in front of you and raise the opposite leg at the same time. Hold for a second and then swap to the opposite arm and leg. Repeat, for as many reps as possible.

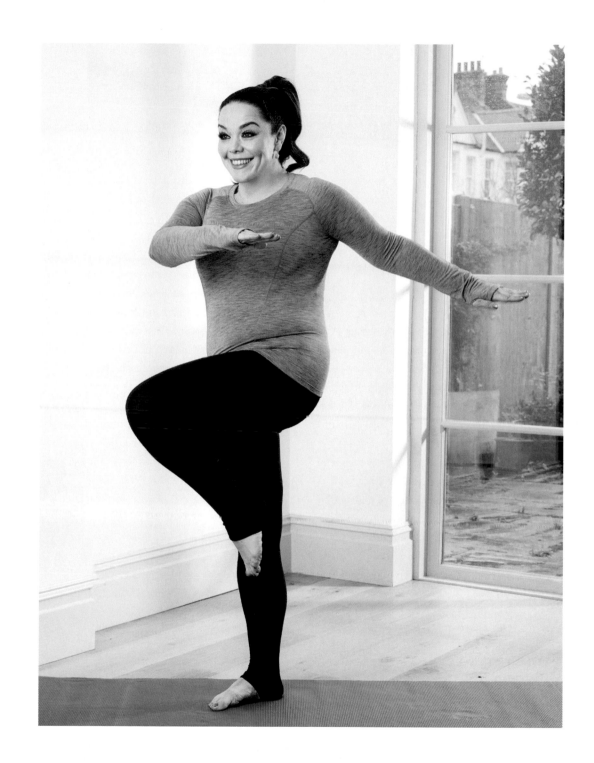

THE KITCHEN WORKOUT

Make the most of cooking time with this mini cardio blast.

1. Grab a couple of tins of food and perform weighted jabs (punches to the front) keeping your hands at chin height. Then twist the hips and punch with the opposite arm as fast as possible.

2. Keeping hold of your tins of food, lower your arms to your sides and then raise them laterally from the side of your body to shoulder height (like wings). Next stretch your arms out in front and then lower to the side in one long flowing movement and repeat.

3. Step into a lunge position with both legs bent and your chest and head up. Grab a large carton of milk with a handle (make sure the lid is secure!) and pass it through and around your legs in a figure-of-eight motion, keeping your stomach tightly held in.

4. Stand up straight and place both hands behind your ears. Raise one knee and reach down to it with your opposite elbow in a twisting motion.

Tense and squeeze your stomach muscles in and then repeat on the other side.

5. Place your hands on your kitchen worktop, shoulder width apart, and shuffle your legs back so you are in a standing plank position. Lower your chest down towards the worktop, keeping your stomach pulled in tightly. Press your body back up to the starting position and repeat.

6. Turn around to face away from the counter and again place your hands on the kitchen worktop. Shuffle your legs forward so they are around a metre away (or whatever feels comfortable). Straighten and lock your arms, raise on to tiptoes and arch your back. Hold for 5 seconds so you can feel the tension in the back of your upper arms. Then, keeping your arms locked and staying on tiptoes, slowly bend your knees to a 90° angle. Hold for 5 seconds, clenching your buttocks. Raise yourself back to a standing position and repeat.

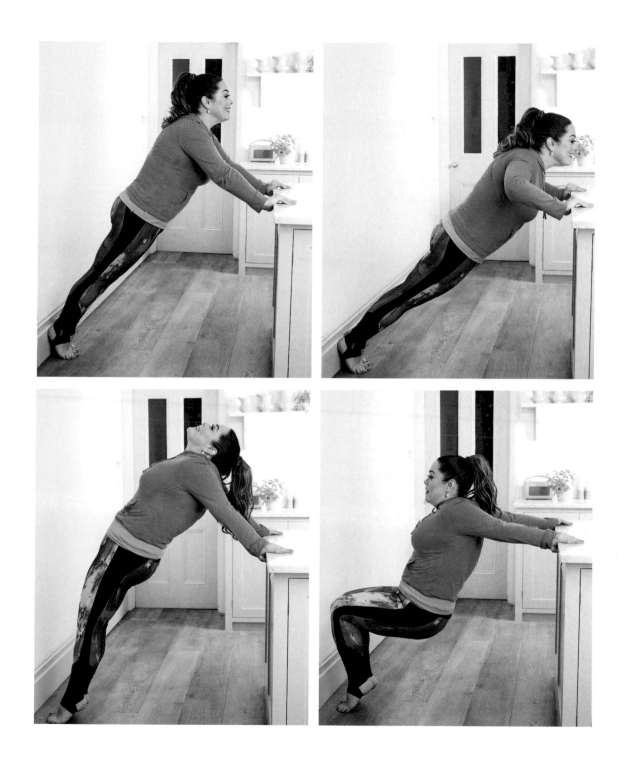

THE STAIRCASE WORKOUT

This is such a brilliant way to exercise in the comfort of your own home.

1. Walk up and down your stairs to warm up the body and increase your heart rate.

2. Stand at the bottom of your staircase facing away from it. Try to squat low enough so that your bum either nearly touches or does touch the first or second step. Make sure your heels stay on the floor and you tense your legs and bum at all times.

3. Kneel about two feet away from the bottom of your staircase and place your hands on either the first or second step (the first step is harder, the second step is easier). Lower your chest to your hands and then press back up while holding your stomach in. Eventually build up to a full press-up with your legs stretched out straight behind you.

4. Place your hands on the first or second step of your staircase (the first step is harder, the second step is easier) and stretch your legs out behind you. Raise one knee to your chest and then do the same on the other side. As you progress, move your legs faster, until you're essentially doing a running motion.

5. Lie at the bottom of your staircase with your bum a foot away from the first step and place your heels on the second or third step (the second is harder and the third easier) with your knees and feet slightly apart. Stretch your arms out in front of you with one palm on top of the other and try to touch the step in between your feet. Pull your arms back in line with your head but don't let your body go all the way to the floor. This way you'll maintain tension in your mid-section at all times.

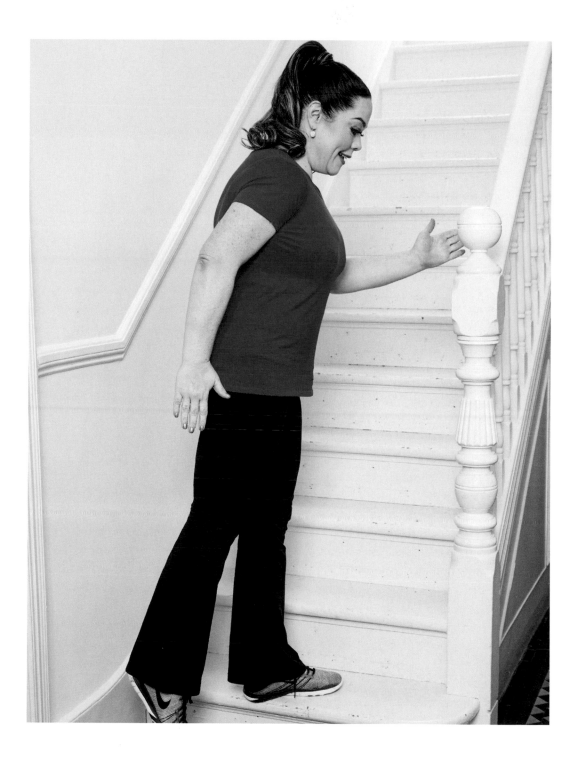

THE TV WORKOUT

Well, if you're going to exercise, why not do it in front of the soaps?

1. Stand in front of the TV with your knees together. Squat a quarter of the way down to the floor and then stand back up, making sure you don't lock your knees when you straighten up. Perform as many mini squats as you can at a fast pace.

2. Stand facing away from the back of your sofa. Slide your body down until your upper back is resting against it. Keep your legs bent in front of you, a couple of feet apart, with your heels only just touching the floor. Raise your hips as high as they will go and pause and tense your bum for a couple of seconds before lowering back down in a controlled manner.

3. Sit at the very front of your sofa, with your arms bent and palms placed flat on the seat area. Either stretch your legs out straight in front of you or bend your legs (bent legs is the easier option). Straighten your arms and lift your bottom off the seat. Bend your arms to 90° and then extend again, tilting your bottom forward and keeping it off the seat throughout. Try to tense and squeeze the back of the top of your arms. This is great for toning bingo wings.

4. Lie on your sofa and place your hands under your lower back. Lock your knees and point your toes, then raise your legs alternately from your hips at 45° angles. Repeat as fast as possible. With this exercise you're targeting the lower stomach.

5. Stand facing your sofa and place your hands on the seat area. Step each leg back and forward alternately as fast as you can. For a harder workout, jump both feet back at once and then jump forward to the sofa.

6. Sit on top of a yoga ball (they are one of my favourite pieces of exercise equipment). Either put your hands behind your head (harder), on the ball (easier), or place one hand against a wall if you need more balance (easier still!). Hold your stomach in and roll your hips to the right and make a small circle. Repeat on the left-hand side. As you become more confident make the circles bigger.

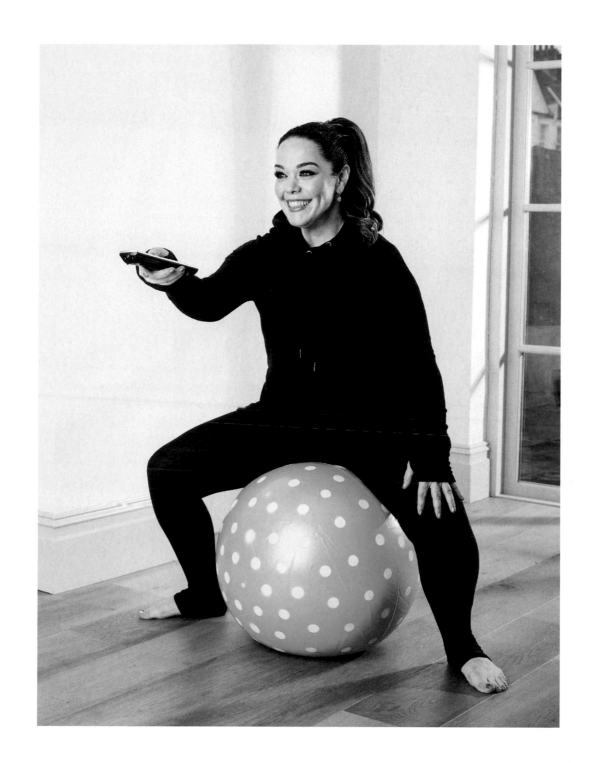

THE ULTIMATE TUMMY TONER

Get fab abs!

1. Lie down on the floor and bend your legs, keeping your feet on the floor and your knees together. Place your fingers on your temples. Raise your head to your knees and then lower, keeping the movement controlled.

2. Stay lying down and place your hands under your lower back for support. Keep your legs locked straight and your toes pointed away. Raise your legs up to a 90° angle and try to raise your bum off the floor slightly at the top of the rep. Tense your abs and then lower your legs in a controlled manner, making sure you don't slam your heels on to the floor.

3. Lie flat on the floor, place your fingers on your temples, bend your legs and bring your knees up to your chest. Reach your hands past your knees while tensing the stomach, and then lower your head and legs back down at the same time. To make it harder, keep your hands on your temples and touch your knees with your elbows.

4. While still lying down, keep your feet flat to the floor with your legs bent and knees together. Place your fingers on the front of your thighs and then slide your hands up your legs and try to touch the top of your knees. Repeat, keeping your head and shoulders off the floor so your stomach stays tense.

5. Finally, lie flat on the floor, raise your head and shoulders off the ground and stretch your arms out in front of you. Raise your legs around 6 inches off the ground and pull in your stomach. Hold for 10–20 seconds and then lower back to the starting position.

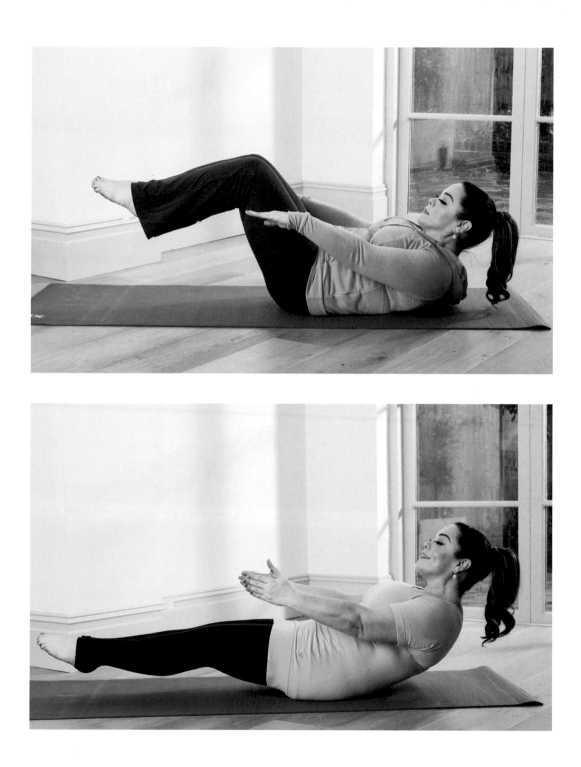

THE LEGS AND BUM WORKOUT

With this one you'll have buns of steel in no time.

1. Warm up by skipping for 5–10 minutes using a HIIT technique – skip slowly for a minute, then fast for a minute, then slowly for a minute, and so on. This will loosen up your whole body.

2. Stand with your feet slightly wider than hip-width apart. Keep your heels on the ground and imagine you are about to sit back on to a chair. Keep your head up and lower back tucked in, then lower your bum past your knees for a count of 3 seconds. Pause for 1 second before slowly returning to a standing position. As soon as your legs are straight, squeeze the legs and bum for a count of 2 seconds before starting the next rep.

3. Follow the same instructions as above but this time repeat the movements in a long, flowing motion without the pause/squeezing in between reps.

4. Lie on the floor with your legs bent, palms facing down and feet around 18 inches apart with your toes in the air. Push through your heels and try to raise your hips above your waistline. Pause and squeeze the front of your thighs before slowly lowering your legs back down.

5. Lie on your front with your palms next to your head and your feet 8 inches apart. Raise your torso and legs from the hips at the same time. Pause and squeeze the bum and lower back before slowly lowering back to a lying position.

6. On your hands and knees, raise one knee off the floor and move it towards your chest before kicking the leg back as high as you can. Repeat on the other side.

7. Standing up straight, place a yoga ball between the base of your spine and the wall. Lower your body into a squat position by rolling the ball down the wall. Stay in the squat for 10–20 seconds before rolling slowly back up to the starting position.

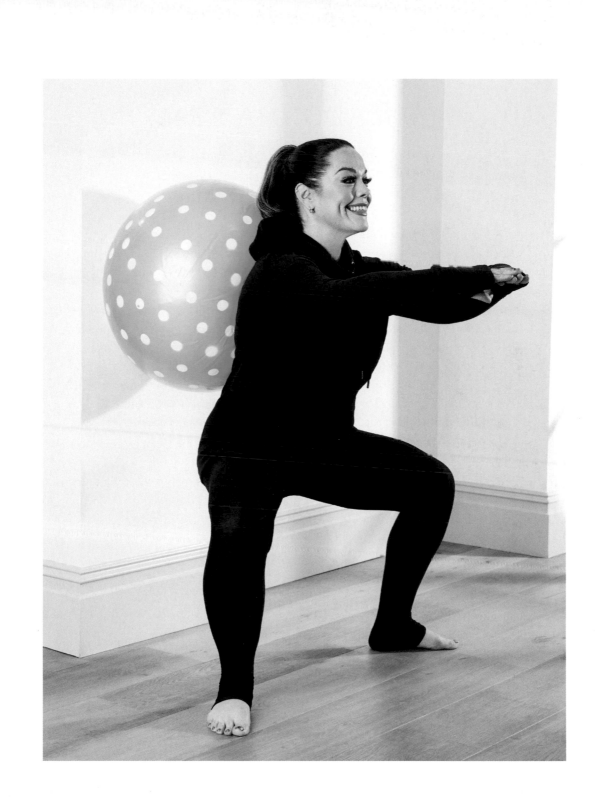

THE MADONNA ARMS WORKOUT

Strong is sexy!

1. Place your palms on a sturdy two-foot-high object (a step, a low bench or a stack of big bulky books will work) with your legs stretched out behind you so your body is flat. Bend and extend the arms so you're doing a mini press-up.

2. While standing, hold a weighted object (for example, a kettle bell or a 2-litre bottle of water) out in front of you and curl your arms up to your chest and back down again in a controlled manner.

3. Still standing and holding the kettle bell or water bottle, stretch your arms above your head. Lower your arms to the back of your head and then straight back up slowly.

4. Hold a dumb-bell in each hand with your arms by the side of your body. Keep your elbows locked and raise your arms up to just above 90°. Lower back down in a controlled manner.

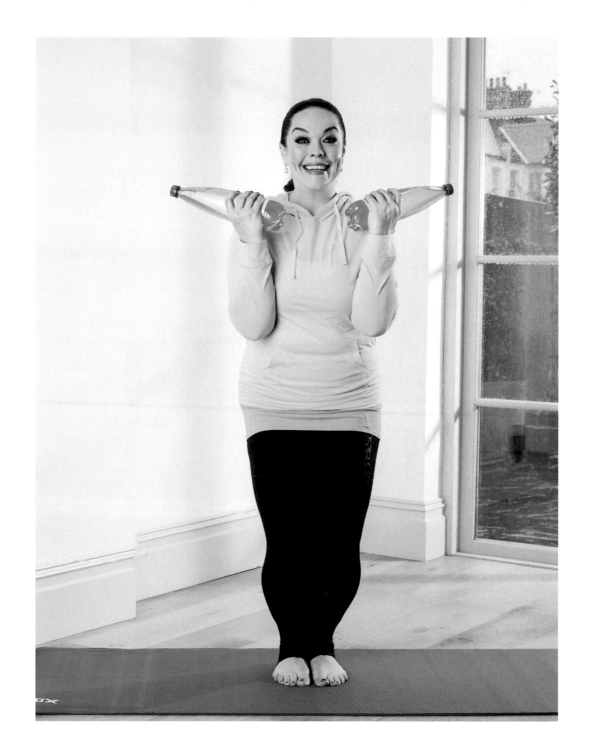

THE SHORT-ON-TIME WORKOUT

Great for when you're in a rush but you still want to work out.

1. Jump your feet out to the side while raising your arms at the same time so you're doing an energetic star jump. Jump your feet back in and lower your arms, staying on your tiptoes, and repeat as fast as you can.

2. Lie down and place your hands under your bum. Raise your head and shoulders off the ground before raising your legs. Keep your feet together, your legs straight and toes pointed away. Hold for 30 seconds.

3. Get into a plank position so you're resting on your elbows with your body straight. Push up into a press-up position, with your arms straight, then back down again while holding in your stomach.

4. Stand with your heels together and feet pointed out. Jump or step both feet out to a squatting position and lean over to one side and try to touch the floor with your hand. Jump or step back to the middle and repeat on the other side.

5. Place your hands on the floor and raise your bum up towards the ceiling while keeping your legs straight. Bring one knee in towards your chest and then straighten the leg again. Swap legs and repeat for several reps as fast as you can.

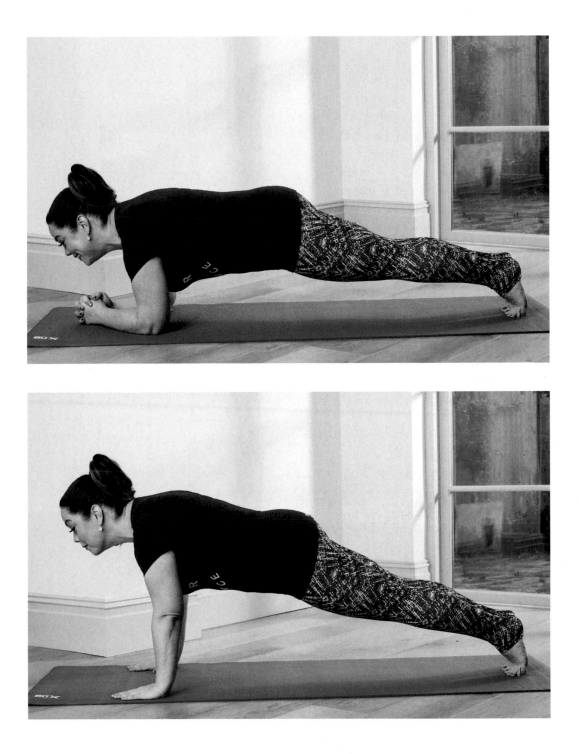

THE HARDCORE WORKOUT

For when you're ready to ramp things up.

1. Bend down so your hands and feet are on the floor and crawl back and forth across the floor keeping your knees off the ground for as long as possible. Take a break and go again!

2. Lie down flat on the floor. Pull yourself up to a standing position using your stomach muscles as much as possible. Jump up keeping your body straight, and then lower yourself back to a lying position. Repeat as many times as possible.

3. Lie down on your back with your feet on the floor and your knees bent and together and place your fingers on your temples. Raise your head to your knees and then lower your head back down. Repeat as many times – and as quickly – as possible.

4. Lower yourself into a squat position and place your hands on the floor in front of you. Jump both legs back so they are straight and hold for a few seconds. Jump the legs back in, stand up and repeat as many times as possible.

5. Hold a plank for between 30 seconds and 1 minute, keeping your stomach taut. Repeat 3 or 4 times. When you're ready to take things to the next level, incorporate a side plank on each arm, holding for between 30 seconds and 1 minute on each side.

6. Sit on the floor and lean your torso back at a 45° angle. Bend your knees and raise your feet very slightly off the floor so you're balancing on your bottom. Hold a kettle bell or a 2-litre bottle of water in front of your chest and twist your torso to the right-hand side so your arms are parallel with the floor. Return to the centre and repeat on the left-hand side. Do this as many times as you can in 30 seconds.

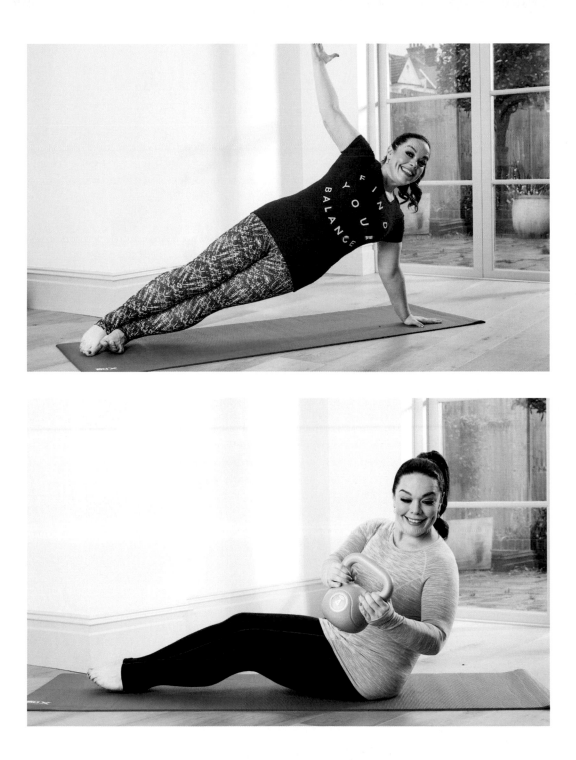

THE PARK WORKOUT

The ultimate way to exercise for free.

You can mix and match the different circuits however you like. The 3-3-3 is a great way to finish, or just do it on its own whenever you need to keep things quick and simple.

1. The legs circuit:
   Begin with a brisk walk around the park
   Do 15 squats
   Jog around the park
   Do 20 lunges
   Run around the park

2. The abs circuit:
   Do a brisk walk around the park
   Do 15 sit-ups
   Jog around the park
   Do 20 leg raises
   Run around the park
   Hold a plank for at least 30 seconds

3. The arms circuit:
   Do a brisk walk around the park
   Do 15 press-ups
   Jog around the park
   Do 15 tricep dips
   Run around the park
   Hold a plank for at least 30 seconds

4. The 3-3-3:
   Walk briskly for 3 minutes
   Jog for 3 minutes
   Run for 3 minutes
   Rest for 3 minutes
   Repeat twice more

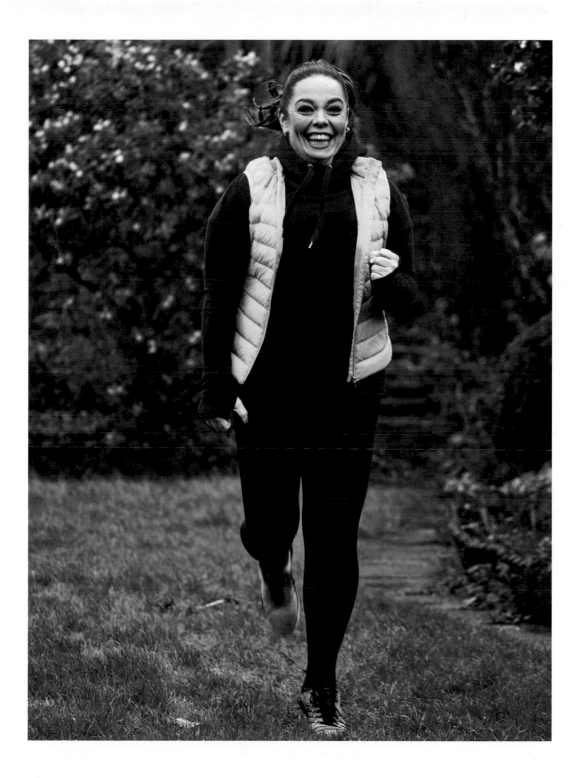

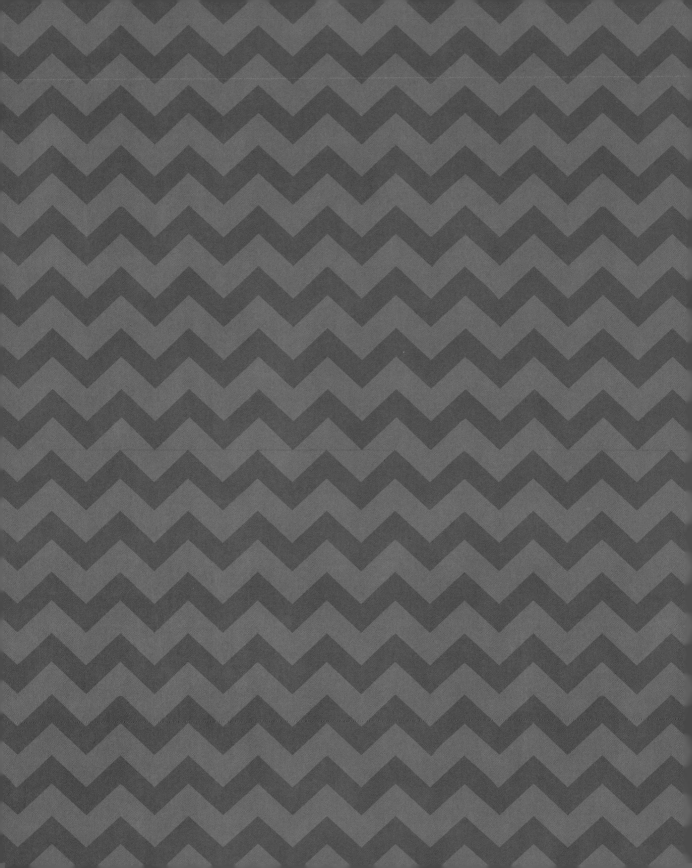

CHAPTER 7

Food Glorious Food

Quick Meals

10-15 MINUTES

SPICY MEXICAN OMELETTE

Spice up your breakfast or lunch with this easy to make, protein-packed taste sensation. Or if you prefer your food less spicy, just leave out the jalapeño chilli.

Serves 1

1 tsp olive oil

1 small red onion, diced

Half a green pepper, deseeded and diced

1 jalapeño chilli, finely chopped (if you can't get jalapeños, then a regular green chilli will be just fine)

2 medium eggs

5g fresh coriander, roughly chopped

1 tomato, diced

Sea salt and freshly ground black pepper

Heat a non-stick frying pan over a medium-high heat and add the olive oil. Tip the pan so the oil coats the base of the pan. Add the diced onion and green pepper and cook for 5 minutes. The onion should be starting to turn golden and the pepper softening. Add the jalapeño and cook for another minute.

Turn the heat right down under the pan and crack the eggs into a jug. Add the coriander, and a little seasoning if you like, and beat well with a fork. Tip the egg mix into the frying pan and use a spoon to lift the vegetables so the egg gets all around and under everything – make sure it coats the whole base of the frying pan. Sprinkle the tomato over the top of the omelette and then after about 1½ minutes, when the egg is largely set, carefully lift the omelette from one side and fold it in half.

Slide on to a plate and eat straight away.

Per serving 226 cals | 15g protein | 12g fat (3g saturates) | 12g carbs (10g total sugars) | 5g fibre

BUCKWHEAT PORRIDGE
WITH ORANGE AND CINNAMON

This is one of my ultimate morning go-tos, and the flavours always remind me of Christmas (even in summer!). Supermarkets sell a wide range of nut milks these days, but if you can't find cashew milk, you can use almond milk instead (which tends to be sold a bit more widely).

Serves 1

40g buckwheat flakes
1 tsp cinnamon
100ml water
100ml cashew milk, unsweetened
1 orange, peeled and cut into segments
1 tbsp runny honey

Tip the buckwheat flakes and cinnamon into a small saucepan and give a little shake to mix them together. Add the water and cashew milk and stir everything together. Start with 100ml of water, but feel free to add more if you like a looser porridge.

Place the pan over a medium-high heat and stir as it slowly comes up to the boil. Then reduce the heat and cook for 3–4 minutes, stirring regularly.

Pour the porridge out into a bowl, top with the orange slices and drizzle over the honey.

Per serving 261 cals | 8g protein | 2g fat (0g saturates) | 50g carbs (24g total sugars) | 1g fibre

CELERIAC AND APPLE SOUP
WITH CHILLI OATCAKES

Just trust me on this one. I know celeriac is a very odd-looking vegetable but it's got a really delicious nutty, slightly sweet flavour. Apple in soup may sound surprising, but you've got to try it. Oatcakes are one of my favourite snacks, and they make the perfect bread substitute. I love the chilli ones, but if you can't find them, plain oatcakes are great too.

Makes 4 portions

1 tsp olive oil
1 onion, diced
2 sticks of celery, diced
10g sage, roughly chopped
1.25 litres fresh vegetable stock, brought to the boil
500g celeriac, peeled and diced
2 large Bramley apples, peeled, cored and diced
Sea salt and freshly ground black pepper
2 chilli oatcakes, to serve

Heat the oil in a large saucepan over a medium-high heat. Add the onion and celery and cook for 3 minutes, stirring often so nothing burns. Add the sage and stir for 20 seconds until you can smell it cooking.

Add the hot stock, followed by all the celeriac and apple. Try to make sure the chopped celeriac and apples are roughly the same size (around 1cm dice) so that everything cooks quickly.

Bring the stock back to the boil and simmer everything for 8–10 minutes, until the celeriac is tender and the apples are broken down. Remove the pan from the heat and use a stick blender/blender/food processor – whatever you have – to blitz everything together into a smooth soup. Have a quick taste and add a little salt and lots of pepper. This is a thick soup, so if you like it thinner just add a little more stock while you are blitzing it.

Serve with the chilli oatcakes on the side.

Lisa's tip: Allow any leftover soup to cool down to room temperature before dividing into portions in airtight storage containers. Once it has fully cooled, you can keep the soup in the fridge for 2–3 days, or freeze for up to 3 months.

Per serving 176 cals | 5g protein | 5g fat (1g saturates) | 23g carbs (17g total sugars) | 11g fibre

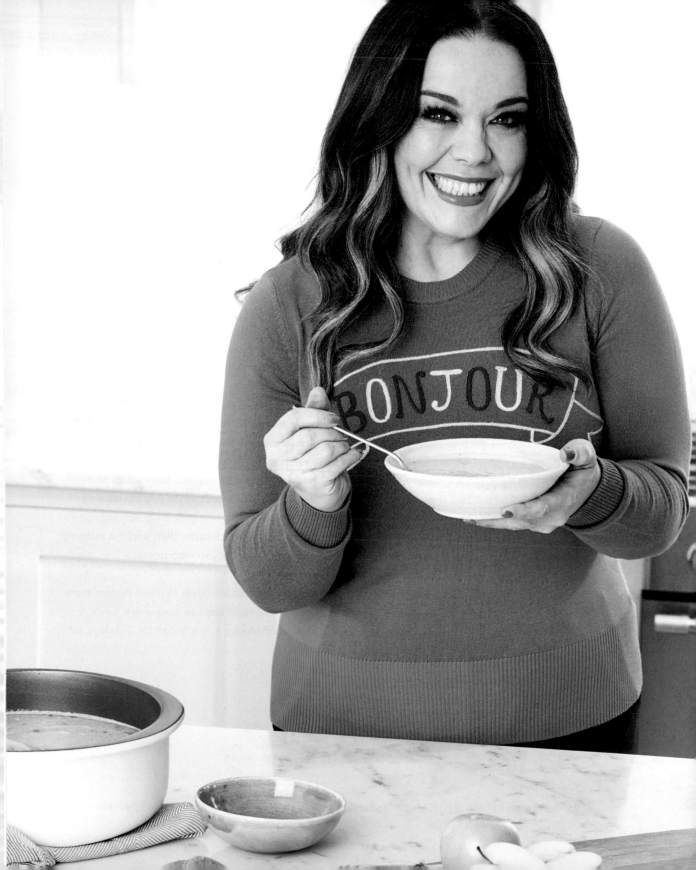

COURGETTE AND GREEN PEPPER PAD THAI

Who'd have thought you could eat a takeaway favourite like pad Thai when you're trying to lose weight? I won't lie, the delicious toasted peanuts are one of the things I love most about this dish. A spiralizer makes light work of prepping the veg (as I mention on page 142, you can pick one up online for less than a tenner), but if you don't have one just slice the courgette into ribbons using a vegetable peeler and cut the green pepper into very skinny strips, and cook them for a little less time than the recipe states.

Serves 2

1 tbsp olive oil

1 red chilli, finely chopped

20g fresh coriander, roughly chopped

2 medium eggs, beaten

2 courgettes, spiralized to make wide, flat noodles

2 green peppers, deseeded and spiralized to make wide, flat noodles

2 tbsp fish sauce

2 tbsp oyster sauce

2 garlic cloves, finely grated

200g beansprouts

40g toasted peanuts, for topping

Juice and zest of 1 lime, to serve

Red chilli and fresh coriander (optional), finely chopped, to serve

Heat the oil in a large wok over a medium-high heat. Add the chilli and coriander and cook for 1 minute. Push everything to one side in the pan and add the beaten eggs to the clear space. Use a spoon or spatula to scramble the eggs really quickly (it shouldn't take more than 1 minute), then incorporate the chilli and coriander.

Add the courgette and pepper noodles to the pan. Cook for 3 minutes, tossing the pan regularly to cook the noodles evenly and mix everything together.

Add the fish sauce, oyster sauce and garlic and toss to coat for 1–2 minutes. The two sauces will reduce quickly in the heat and coat the vegetables, at which point add the beansprouts and cook for another 2 minutes.

Remove from the heat, divide between two bowls and top with the toasted peanuts. Grate over the lime zest and squeeze over the juice.

You could serve with some extra red chilli or coriander on top if you like.

Per serving 347 cals | 21g protein | 21g fat (4g saturates) | 16g carbs (9g total sugars) | 7g fibre

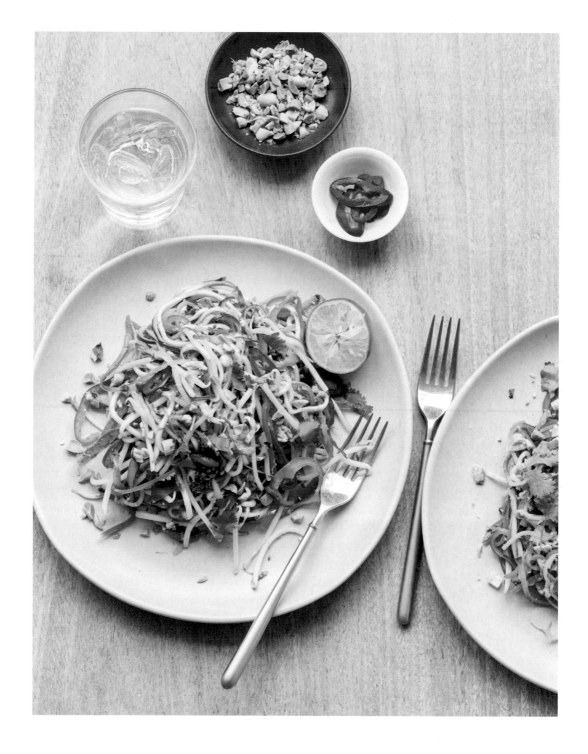

VEGGIE NOODLE STIR-FRY

This is so easy to make and brilliantly tasty and crunchy, not to mention colourful. A spiralizer makes prepping vegetables so quick: you literally just top and tail any vegetable, push it on to or into the spiralizer and turn – 30 seconds later you have a mound of amazing vegetable noodles. You can get one online for less than a tenner (in fact mine cost just a few pounds!), and it's a great little purchase if you love your veggies.

Serves 2

1 tbsp toasted sesame oil

2 garlic cloves, finely grated

2cm piece of ginger, finely grated

1 sweet potato, peeled and spiralized

1 courgette, spiralized

1 yellow pepper, deseeded and spiralized

1 orange pepper, deseeded and spiralized

1 green pepper, deseeded and spiralized

1 tbsp sriracha (more if you like the heat)

1 tbsp runny honey

10g fresh coriander, roughly chopped

20g toasted sesame seeds, for topping

1 lime, cut into wedges, to serve

Heat the oil in a large wok over a medium-high heat. Add the garlic and ginger. Stir quickly for 30 seconds before adding all the spiralized vegetables. Toss the vegetables in the garlic, ginger and oil to coat them, and keep them moving for 3–4 minutes.

Mix the sriracha and honey together in a small bowl and add to the pan. Stir the noodles until they are all coated.

Turn off the heat and add the coriander, giving the pan one last shake to incorporate.

Divide the noodles between two bowls and top each with half of the toasted sesame seeds. Serve with a lime wedge for a citrus kick.

Per serving 252 cals | 5g protein | 8g fat (2g saturates) | 35g carbs (20g total sugars) | 9g fibre

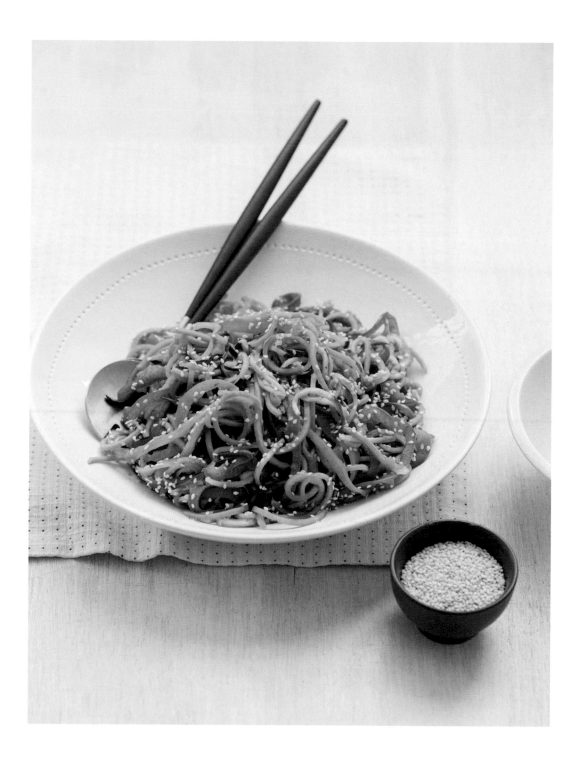

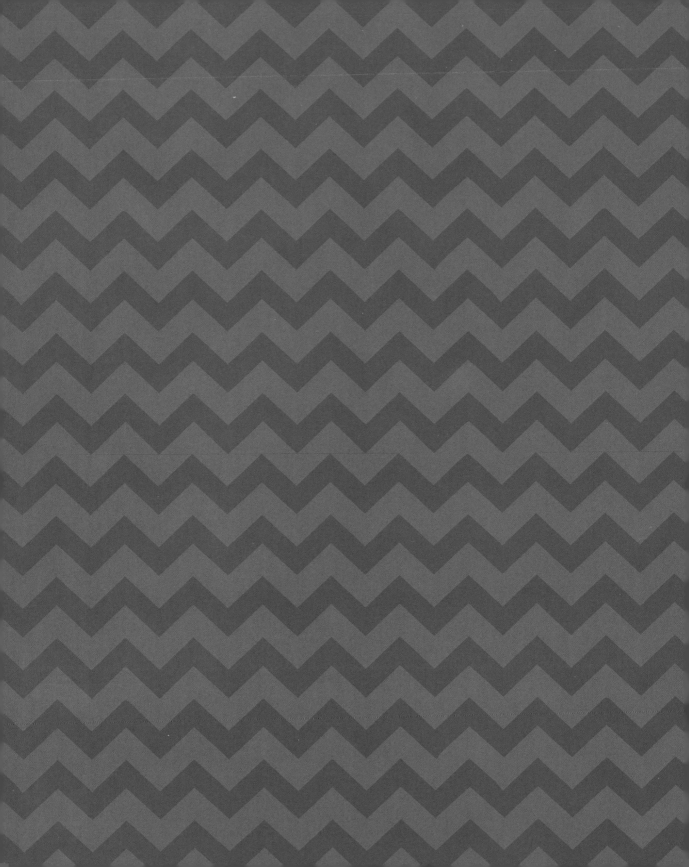

Recipes to up Your Game

20-30 MINUTES

ITALIAN-STYLE CHICKEN TRAY BAKE

This dish is ridiculously easy. You literally bung everything into a roasting tin and it comes out looking and smelling like you've been slaving in the kitchen for hours. Minimal washing-up too!

Serves 2

4 chicken thighs on the bone, skinless

3 tomatoes, quartered

1 aubergine, cubed

1 courgette, cut into chunks

1 yellow pepper, deseeded and cut into chunks

4 garlic cloves, thinly sliced

1 tbsp olive oil

1 tbsp dried oregano

50g mixed olives, pitted

1 tbsp balsamic vinegar

Sea salt and freshly ground black pepper

5g fresh basil leaves, to garnish

Preheat the oven to 190°C/Fan 170°C/Gas 5.

Line a roasting tin with non-stick baking paper and place the chicken thighs in it. Add the tomatoes, aubergine, courgette, pepper and garlic. Drizzle over the olive oil and sprinkle over the oregano. Season with salt and black pepper. Shake the roasting tin to coat everything in the oil and seasoning.

Place the roasting tin in the hot oven for 15 minutes. Remove the tin, turn the vegetables and add the olives. Return to the oven for another 8–10 minutes (or until the chicken thighs are cooked through).

Remove the tray from the oven and drizzle over the balsamic vinegar. Garnish with the basil leaves before serving.

Per serving 426 cals | 34g protein | 26g fat (6g saturates) | 11g carbs (10g total sugars) | 8g fibre

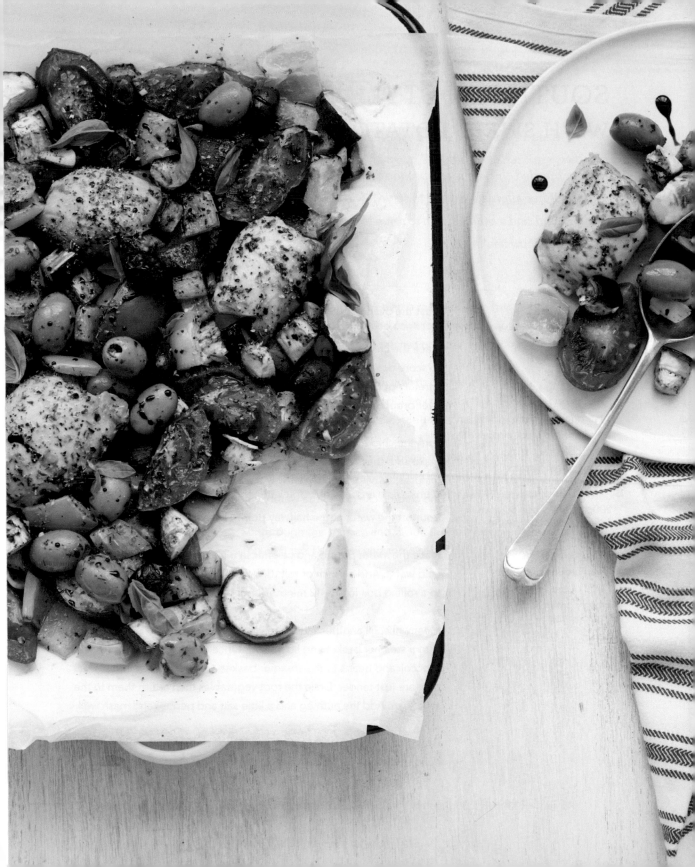

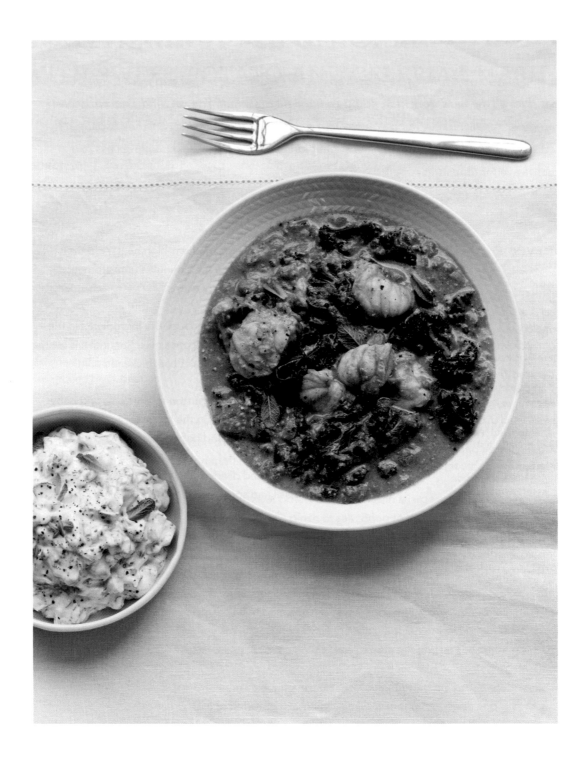

MONKFISH AND KALE TIKKA MASALA
WITH LOW-FAT RAITA

The first time I tasted this I thought I'd died and gone to heaven. Forget takeaway tikka masala, this is your new and guilt-free Friday-night dinner! Monkfish is a meaty fish, so it works well in a curry, though I've also made this using salmon fillets and it tasted every bit as good.

Serves 2

1 tsp olive oil

1 red onion, diced

1 red chilli, finely chopped (optional)

3 garlic cloves, finely grated

3cm piece of ginger, peeled and grated

2 tbsp tikka masala spice paste

2 tbsp ground almonds

1 x 400g tin chopped tomatoes

1 x 400g tin low-fat coconut milk

250g monkfish loin (or salmon fillets)

200g kale, tough stalks removed

For the raita:

150g low-fat yoghurt

10g fresh mint leaves, roughly chopped

Quarter of a cucumber, seeds removed and diced

Sea salt and freshly ground black pepper

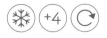

Heat the oil in a large saucepan over a medium-high heat. Add the onion and chilli. Cook for 5–6 minutes until they have softened and the onion has started to turn golden brown.

Add the garlic and ginger and cook for another 30 seconds, stirring frequently so nothing burns. Add the spices and ground almonds and mix well to coat everything in the pan before adding the chopped tomatoes and coconut milk.

Simmer the sauce for 15 minutes and allow to thicken. Stir occasionally to stop anything catching on the bottom of the pan.

In the meantime, cut the monkfish loin into big chunks (around 3cm slices). Once the sauce has thickened, add the kale and stir through. It should start to wilt quite quickly; give it 3 minutes and then carefully add the monkfish.

Allow it all to cook together for 4–5 minutes, over a very low heat, while you make the raita, which is really quick. Mix the yoghurt, mint leaves and cucumber together in a little bowl along with the seasoning.

Then all that's left to do is serve the curry alongside the mint raita.

Per serving 515 cals | 35g protein | 29g fat (14g saturates) | 25g carbs (21g total sugars) | 9g fibre

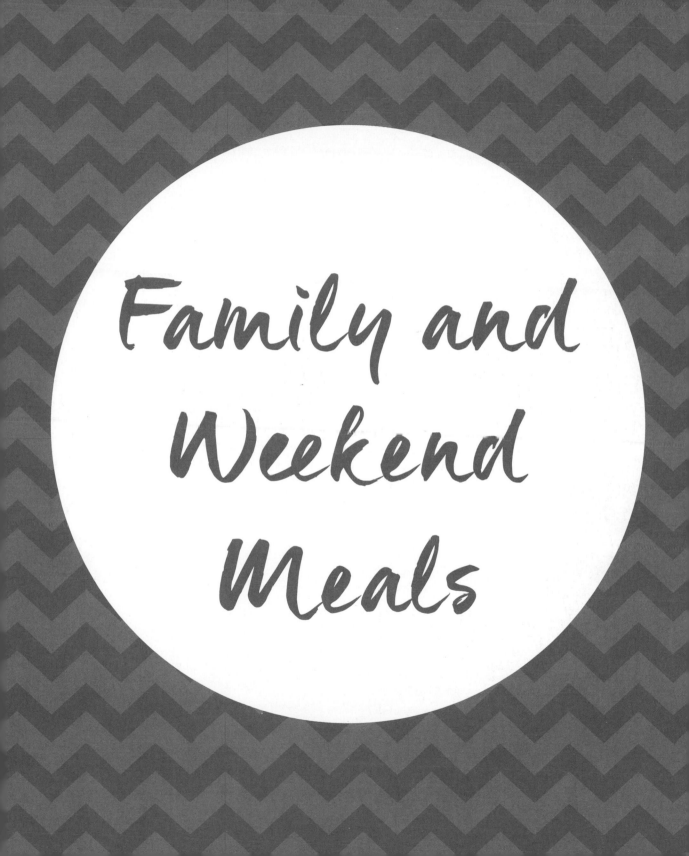

Family and Weekend Meals

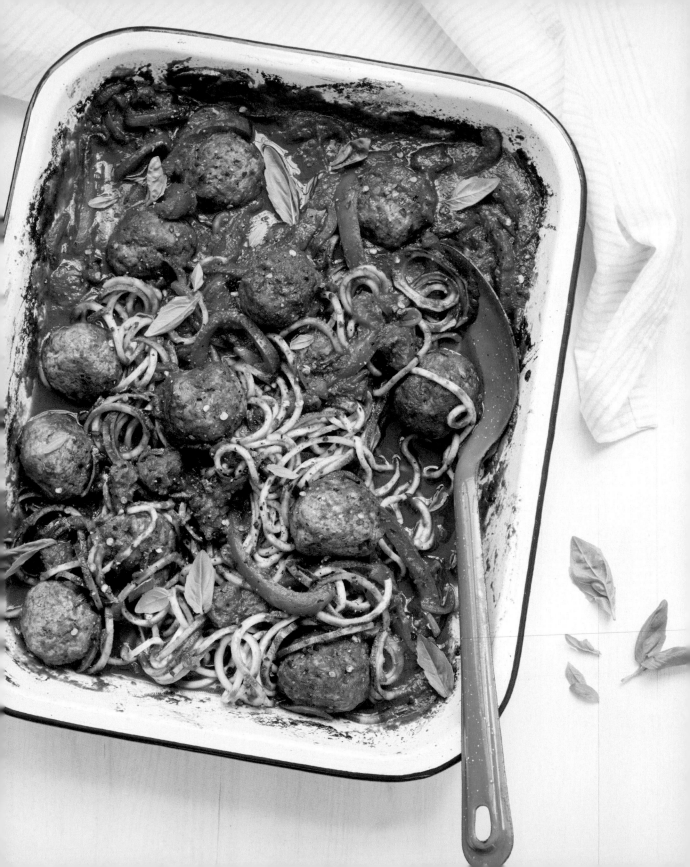

TURKEY MEATBALL TRAY BAKE

If you've got people coming round for dinner no one is going to complain when you serve this. It's a real crowd-pleaser. Turkey mince makes for much healthier meatballs than classic beef ones, because it contains a lot less fat. If you don't want to spiralize your courgettes, you could slice them into long ribbons with a vegetable peeler, and give them a little less time in the steamer.

Serves 4

500g turkey mince
1 tbsp dried oregano
1 tbsp smoked paprika
1 tsp garlic powder
100g cooking chorizo
2 red onions, thinly sliced
1 red pepper, deseeded and sliced
500g passata
4 courgettes, spiralized
10g fresh basil leaves, roughly chopped
Sea salt and freshly ground black pepper
2 tsp chilli flakes (optional), for topping

Preheat the oven to 200°C/Fan 180°C/Gas 6.

Place the turkey mince in a mixing bowl along with the oregano, paprika and garlic powder. Add a little seasoning if you like at this point, then mix everything together well with your hands. Divide the mince into 12 even amounts and shape into balls. Pop them into a large non-stick roasting tin as you do them.

Peel the skin off the cooking chorizo, tear into bite-size pieces and scatter them around the turkey meatballs. Place the roasting tin in the oven for 10 minutes. Remove the tin from the oven and add the onions and pepper. Stir everything around in the oil from the chorizo and return the tray to the oven for another 10 minutes. Remove the tray again and add the passata and some seasoning, making sure everything is well coated in the tomato sauce. Return to the oven for another 10 minutes.

While this is finishing off in the oven, fill a saucepan with 5cm of water and bring to the boil with a steamer basket and lid on top. Once the water is boiling, add the courgetti to the basket and cook for 2–3 minutes, until just softening. Then drain and shake off any excess water.

Remove the roasting tin from the oven and add the courgetti to it. Gently toss or mix everything together, adding the chopped basil as you go. Divide into four portions and top with a sprinkle of chilli flakes if you like.

Per serving 414 cals | 47g protein | 17g fat (6g saturates) | 15g carbs (13g total sugars) | 6g fibre

BEAN BURGERS AND SWEET POTATO WEDGES

Who says you can't eat burgers and wedges when you're on a diet? These veggie delights make you feel like you're eating out when you're eating in. No buns, though, please – this recipe is deliberately bread-free.

Serves 4

2 carrots (150g), peeled and cut into 1cm pieces

2 parsnips (150g), peeled and cut into 1cm pieces

2 x 400g tins kidney beans, drained

20g fresh coriander, finely chopped

1 tsp ground cumin

½ tsp cayenne pepper (optional)

400g sweet potatoes, washed and cut into wedges

1 tbsp olive oil

1 tsp dried oregano

8 lettuce leaves

1 tomato, sliced

1 avocado, sliced

Sea salt and freshly ground black pepper

Preheat the oven to 200°C/Fan 180°C/Gas 6.

Pop the carrots and parsnips into a saucepan and cover with cold water. Place on the hob over a medium-high heat and bring the water up to the boil. Keep the water at a rolling boil until the vegetables are cooked through – this should take around 10–12 minutes.

Drain the vegetables and return them to the saucepan. Add one tin of kidney beans and mash into a thick paste. Add the second tin of beans, the coriander, cumin, cayenne pepper (if using) and some seasoning, and fold everything into the paste until you have a firm and chunky mix. Divide into four and shape into hearty patties. Pop them on to a square of baking paper and put them in the fridge on a chopping board to set for 30 minutes.

Line a baking sheet with baking paper and lay out the sweet potato wedges. Drizzle over the olive oil, oregano and a twist of black pepper.

Take another baking sheet and slide the chilled burgers on to it. Pop both sheets into the oven and cook for 25 minutes, turning the sweet potatoes over halfway through the cooking time.

Lay out four lettuce leaves, top with a bean burger, a slice or two of tomato and avocado and the remaining lettuce leaves, so you have a bread-free burger. Divide the wedges and enjoy burger night!

Per serving 382 cals | 12g protein | 12g fat (2g saturates) | 48g carbs (12g total sugars) | 19g fibre

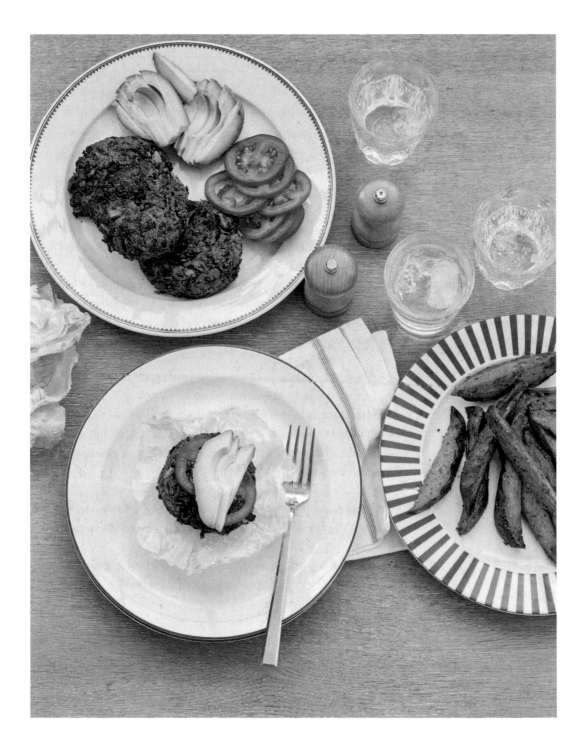

STUFFED BAKED SWEET POTATOES AND POACHED EGGS

I'm cautious about recommending sweet potatoes because too many people dish up sweet potato fries and kid themselves they're healthy. But baked sweet potato is a different matter, and it's so tasty with this delicious black bean and avocado topping. This is another recipe that will keep the whole family happy.

Serves 4

4 sweet potatoes, each
    weighing 150–175g
1 tbsp olive oil
1 onion, diced
2 garlic cloves,
    finely grated
3 tomatoes, chopped
1 x 400g tin black beans,
    drained and rinsed
1 avocado, chopped
10g fresh coriander,
    roughly chopped
1 tbsp white wine vinegar
4 medium eggs (the fresher
    the better, for poaching)
Sea salt and freshly ground
    black pepper

Preheat the oven to 190°C/Fan 170°C/Gas 5.

Scrub the sweet potatoes under running water to make sure they're nice and clean, then pop them on to a baking sheet lined with non-stick baking paper. Place the tray in the hot oven and bake for 35 minutes or until a skewer goes through them easily.

When there is around 15 minutes of cooking time left, place a large deep pan of water over a high heat and bring it to the boil. Meanwhile, heat the olive oil in a frying pan over a medium-high heat. Add the onion and cook for 5 minutes until it just starts to soften.

Add the garlic to the onion and cook for another 30 seconds before adding the chopped tomatoes. Continue cooking and stirring for another 4–5 minutes until the tomatoes have cooked down and made a thick sauce – you don't want it to be watery.

Add the black beans and cook for another 3 minutes to heat through, stirring frequently. Remove from the heat and add the avocado and chopped coriander. Set to one side.

The saucepan of water should be boiling by now. Add the vinegar and reduce the heat so the water is just simmering. Crack two

Per serving 434 cals | 15g protein | 16g fat (3g saturates) | 52g carbs (14g total sugars) | 13g fibre

eggs into two small cups or ramekins. Use a spoon to stir the water round and round; you want to make it spin and create a vortex in the middle. Once the water is spinning, take one of the eggs and quickly tip it in, close to the edge of the pan; the water will pull it around and into the middle of the pan. Quickly add the second egg. Poach for between 2½ and 3 minutes for a runny yolk. Remove and drain on kitchen paper to soak up any water, then repeat for the other two eggs.

Remove the sweet potatoes from the oven and slice lengthways down from the top. Press them open to create space for your filling and divide the bean mixture between them. Top with a poached egg, and season with some salt and pepper.

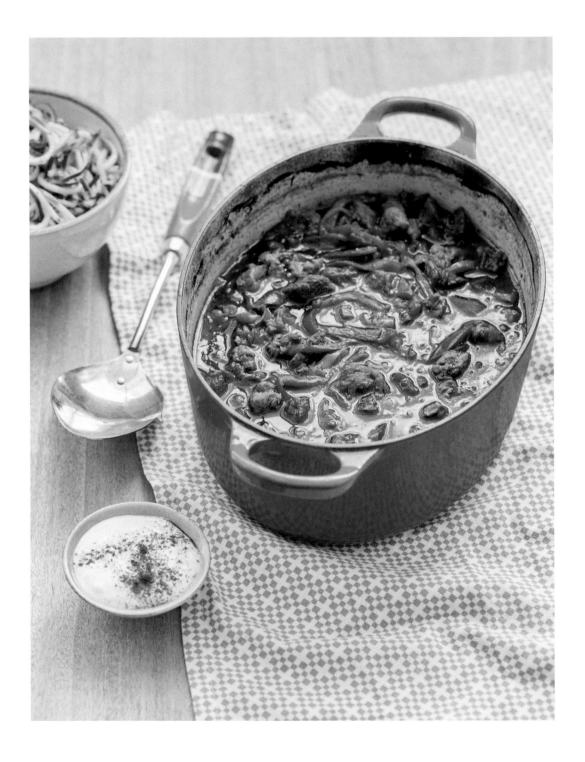

PORK GOULASH

This is another one of those dishes where you can bung everything in together and create something worthy of a MasterChef trophy. It's got a great smoky flavour from the paprika. It does need quite a long time in the oven, so it's not one to do if you're in a hurry. I eat this with courgette noodles, but if you're serving it to the family too, they could have theirs with some couscous.

Serves 4

2 tbsp olive oil

1kg pork shoulder, cut into 3–4cm pieces

2 red onions, thinly sliced

2 red peppers, deseeded and sliced

2 green peppers, deseeded and sliced

2 tbsp tomato purée

2 tbsp sweet smoked paprika

2 garlic cloves, finely grated

1 tbsp dried oregano

1 x 400g tin chopped tomatoes

2 tbsp red wine vinegar

4 courgettes, spiralized

Juice of 1 lemon

10g fresh flat-leaf parsley, roughly chopped

4 tbsp low-fat sour cream

Sea salt and freshly ground black pepper

A sprinkle of paprika, to garnish

Preheat the oven to 170°C/Fan 150°C/Gas 3.

Heat one tablespoon of the olive oil in a large casserole pot over a medium-high heat. Season the meat with a little salt and pepper and fry it in a few batches, adding the meat to the pot and browning it on all sides until golden. Transfer to a dish to one side of you as it cooks and keep handy.

Add the onions and cook for 5 minutes until they too are starting to turn golden brown. Add the peppers, tomato purée, paprika, garlic and oregano. Cook for 1 minute, stirring continuously, to mix everything together. Return the meat to the casserole pot and stir to combine.

Add the tomatoes and red wine vinegar and enough water to cover the meat. Bring everything up to a gentle simmer, then turn off the heat, pop the lid on and place the casserole dish in the oven.

Cook for 90 minutes, stirring halfway through the cooking time. After 90 minutes, remove the lid and cook, uncovered, for a final 30 minutes. Remove the casserole from the oven and allow it to rest while you cook the noodles.

Heat the remaining oil in a large wok and add the courgette noodles. Toss to cook them evenly for 2–3 minutes, until they just start to soften. Turn the heat down and add the lemon juice and parsley. Toss to coat the noodles, then serve immediately with the goulash and a dollop of sour cream. Garnish with a sprinkle of paprika.

Per serving 495 cals | 58g protein | 20g fat (6g saturates) | 18g carbs (16g total sugars) | 7g fibre

FISH TACOS
WITH LETTUCE WRAPS

Arriba! I love a feisty Mexican, and the chilli, paprika and red onions in this recipe will have your tongue doing cartwheels. Making your own spice rub for the fish may seem like added work, but it is the best way to make sure you know what's in it – a lot of supermarket blends have hidden salts and sugars.

Serves 4

1 tsp olive oil
1 tbsp smoked paprika
1 tsp dried oregano
1 tsp chilli flakes
4 x 125g cod fillets
1 cos lettuce, broken
   into leaves
1 red onion, diced
4 tomatoes, diced
2 avocados, diced.
2 red chillis, thinly sliced
10g fresh coriander leaves

Place the oil and spices in a shallow dish and mix well. Add the fish and turn the fillets to coat them in the mix.

Heat a frying pan over a medium-high heat and add the fish to the pan. Cook for 3 minutes, before carefully turning and cooking for another 2 minutes. Remove from the pan and allow to rest for 1 minute.

Take one fillet per serving and use a fork to break it into delicious flakes of fish.

Take a lettuce wrap and add some of the onion, tomato and avocado. Add some of the fish flakes, and top with a few slices of chilli and some coriander leaves.

Per serving 295 cals | 25g protein | 17g fat (4g saturates) | 7g carbs (6g total sugars) | 7g fibre

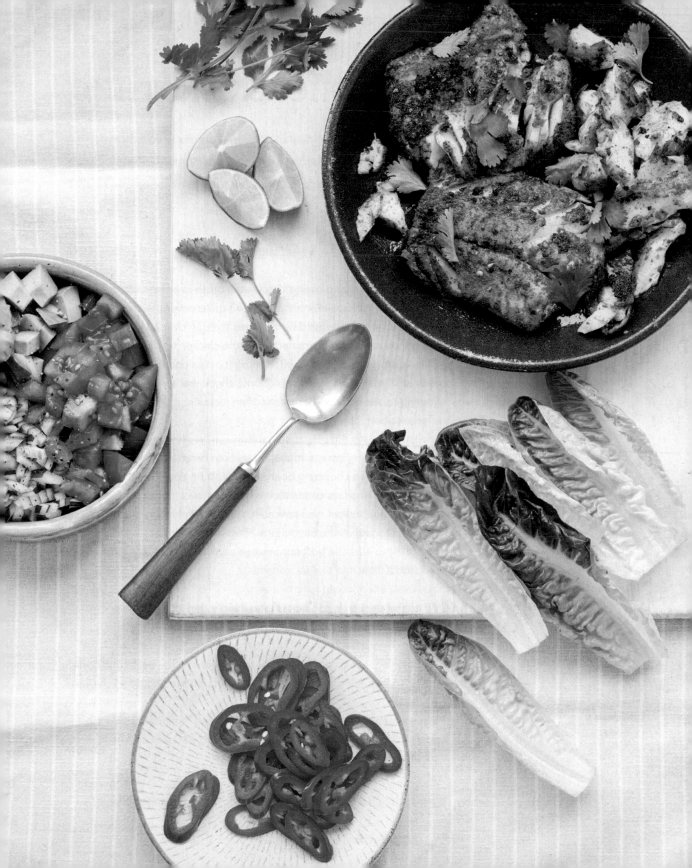

GRILLED HONEY SALMON SALAD
WITH BEETROOT AND PINE NUTS

This recipe is so good. It's an ideal weekend meal for when you have guests round and your friends will thank you for it. The sweet honey glaze is also a great way to make salmon a bit more family-friendly if your kids aren't too sure about fish.

Serves 4

2 tsp olive oil

4 raw beetroot, peeled and cut into 8 wedges

4 tsp clear honey

100g pine nuts

4 skinless salmon fillets

300ml fresh vegetable stock

1 bay leaf

Juice of 2 lemons, freshly squeezed

300g bag mixed salad leaves

Sea salt and freshly ground black pepper

Preheat the oven to 180°C/Fan 160°/Gas 4. Lightly grease a piece of foil with the oil and arrange the beetroot wedges on top. Then close the foil around them to make a sealed parcel. Place the foil parcel on a baking tray and roast in the oven for about 50 minutes or until just soft. Drizzle half the honey over the hot beetroot and toss to coat thoroughly. Season with salt and pepper, then place the beetroot back in the oven and roast, uncovered, for about 10 minutes.

While the beetroot is cooking, heat a frying pan on the hob over a medium heat and add the pine nuts. Toss frequently until they are lightly toasted. Then transfer to a bowl to cool slightly.

Place your salmon fillets in the frying pan and season with black pepper before pouring over the stock. Add the bay leaf and bring gently to the boil with the lid on. Lower the heat and simmer for 8 minutes. Remove the salmon and discard the poaching liquid.

Lightly brush each salmon fillet with the remaining honey, using a brush. Pop under a medium-hot grill, honey side up, skin side down, for 5 minutes and let the fish get some colour. Do not turn the salmon.

Put your salad leaves into a large bowl and dress with lemon juice, then season with salt and pepper. Add the beetroot and toss lightly. Remove the salmon from the grill and, once it's cool enough to handle, flake it into the salad. Finish by sprinkling over the pine nuts.

Per serving 548cals | 34g protein | 39g fat (5g saturates) | 14g carbs (13g total sugars) | 5g fibre

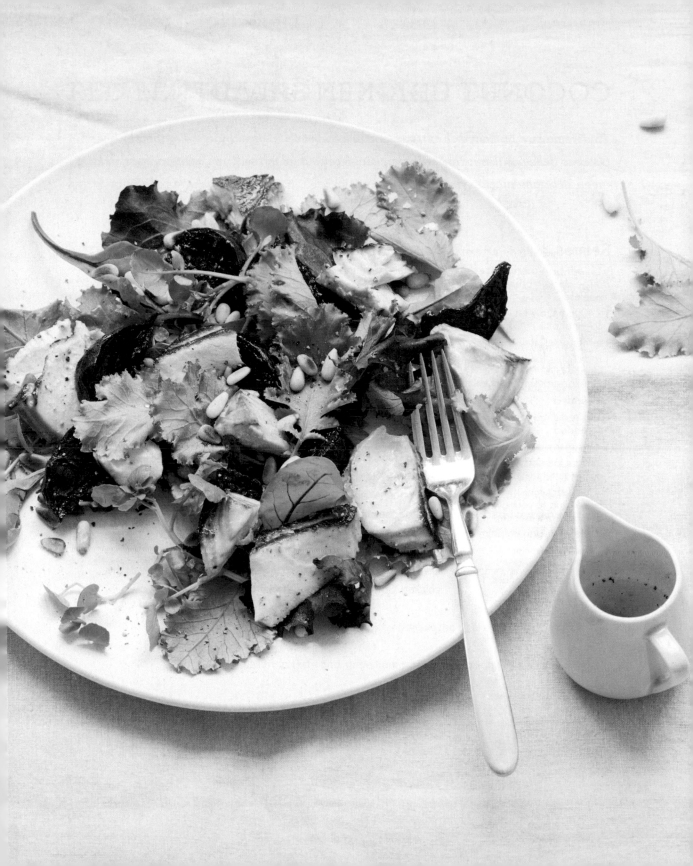

FISH AND CHIPS WITH MINTY PEAS

I never forget my Northern roots! Imagine your mates' surprise when you invite them round for fish and chips. This feels like the ultimate Friday-night treat. You'll love my chips with a difference and my delicious healthy alternative to deep-fried batter! No looking back...

Serves 4

2 large carrots, peeled and cut into chips

2 large parsnips, peeled and cut into chips

1 celeriac, peeled and cut into chips

1 tbsp olive oil

4 x 150g haddock or cod fillets

1 tsp Dijon mustard

Zest of 1 lemon

10g fresh flat-leaf parsley, finely chopped

10g chives, finely chopped

20g Parmesan cheese, finely grated

Sea salt and freshly ground black pepper

For the minty peas:

240g frozen garden peas

10g fresh mint leaves, finely chopped

2 tbsp low-fat crème fraîche

Juice of 1 lemon

Preheat the oven to 200°C/Fan 180°C/Gas 6.

Line a roasting tin with non-stick baking paper. Put all the vegetable chips into the roasting tin and drizzle over the olive oil. Add some seasoning, and then pop them into the hot oven to roast for 25 minutes.

While the chips are cooking, take the four fish fillets and lay them on a baking sheet. Add a little of the mustard to the top of each and spread it over the fish in a thin layer.

In a small bowl put the lemon zest, parsley, chives and Parmesan cheese, and mix well. Divide the herb mix between the four fish fillets and spread it out, pressing it down lightly on to the mustard.

Once the chips have had their first 25 minutes, remove the tray and turn them over. Return them to the oven along with the fish, putting the fish on the higher shelf. Cook everything together for another 8 minutes.

While everything is cooking, bring a saucepan of water to the boil and add the frozen peas. Cook for 5 minutes until tender. Transfer half of them to a food processor or mini-chopper along with the mint leaves and crème fraîche, and blitz until quite smooth. Add the remaining peas and lemon juice and give it a few quick pulses to bring everything together.

Serve up the fish, chips and minty peas between four plates and tuck right in!

Per serving 291 cals | 34g protein | 7g fat (3g saturates) | 17g carbs (11g total sugars) | 10g fibre

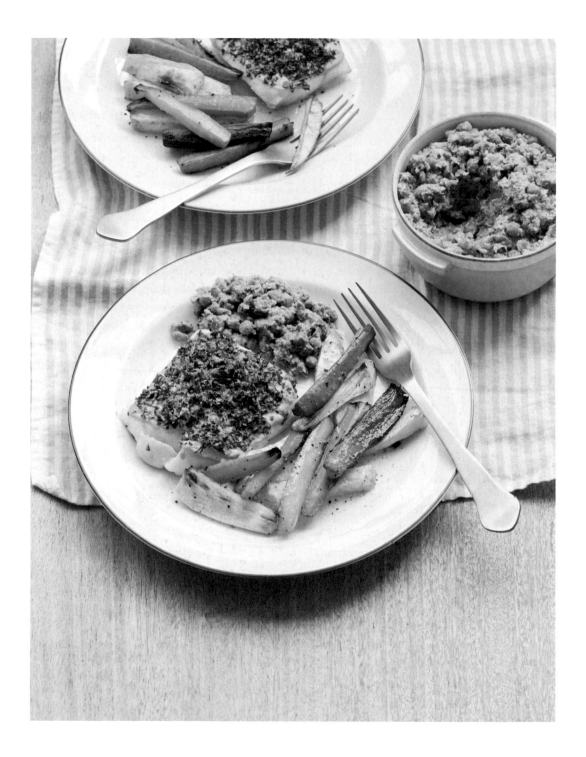

BAKED FALAFEL SALAD

I always assumed falafels were a bit posh and hippie, and not really for me, but I quickly changed my mind when I tried them. They taste amazing and they're so good for eating on the go. It's easy to make your own, and then you know exactly what's gone into them.

Serves 6

2 x 400g tins chickpeas, drained

2 garlic cloves, finely grated

20g fresh flat-leaf parsley, roughly chopped

2 tbsp brown rice flour

1 tsp ground cumin

200g mixed salad leaves

200g roasted red peppers, deseeded and torn into strips

100g cherry tomatoes, halved

1 red onion, thinly sliced

1 avocado, chopped

Sea salt and freshly ground black pepper

Zest of 1 lemon, to garnish

For the dressing:

50g low-fat natural yoghurt

1 tbsp harissa

Juice of 1 lemon

Preheat the oven to 200°C/Fan 180°C/Gas 6.

Place the drained chickpeas, garlic, parsley, brown rice flour, cumin and a little seasoning in a food processor and pulse everything into a coarse paste. You don't want it to be smooth, but chunky.

Take golf ball-sized amounts of the chickpea mix, roll them into balls and place them on a baking sheet covered with non-stick baking paper, leaving a little space between them. Repeat until you have used all the mix – you should have twelve balls.

Place the baking sheet in the oven and bake for 20–25 minutes, until they are golden brown and crisp on the outside.

While the falafels bake, you can make the salad. Put the mixed salad leaves, peppers, tomatoes, onion and avocado into a large bowl and mix well. Transfer to a large serving plate.

Make the dressing by mixing together the yoghurt, harissa and lemon juice. Set to one side.

Top the salad with the baked falafels, and dollop on the dressing. Finish by sprinkling over the lemon zest.

Per serving 306 cals | 13g protein | 12g fat (2g saturates) | 32g carbs (7g total sugars) | 11g fibre

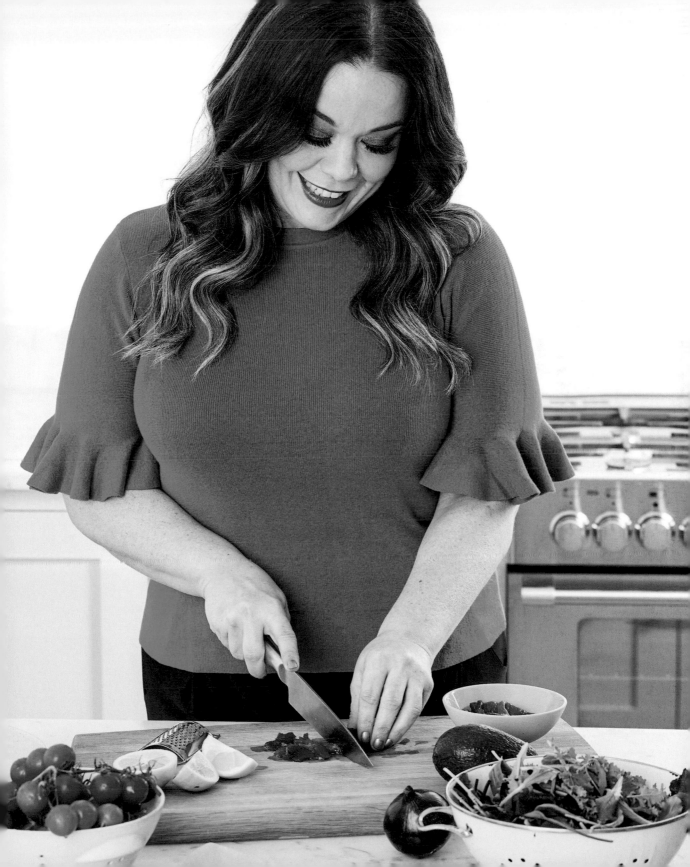

GRIDDLED CHICKEN
WITH SATAY CORN ON THE COB

This is a great dinner for the summer when you want to join in the barbecue without ruining your diet! I absolutely love peanut satay, and this home-made version takes corn on the cob to a whole new level. Just add a handful of green salad leaves to finish the meal off.

Serves 4

4 chicken breasts, skinless
1 tbsp olive oil
4 corn on the cob
4 tbsp crunchy peanut butter
1 tbsp low-salt soy sauce
1 tbsp mirin
2 tbsp cold water
Sea salt and freshly ground black pepper
300g bag green salad leaves, to serve

Take a sheet of baking paper and lay a chicken breast on it. Fold the paper over the top, then take a rolling pin and give the breast a bit of a bash. Don't hit it too hard, as you don't want to break the chicken up. Bash it until it is about 1cm thick all over – this makes it quicker and easier to cook. Repeat with the other three breasts. Place the chicken breasts in a mixing bowl and add the oil and some seasoning. Turn the chicken to coat the flesh evenly.

Bring a large saucepan of water to the boil, and heat a griddle pan over a medium-high heat.

Add the corn to the boiling water and cook for 8 minutes. While this is cooking, add two chicken breasts to the griddle and cook for 4 minutes on each side (checking they are cooked through before removing from the griddle). Repeat for the other two breasts, keeping the cooked chicken warm until you are ready to eat.

While the chicken is on the griddle, mix together the crunchy peanut butter, soy sauce, mirin and the cold water. Mix vigorously until you have a well-blended satay sauce.

Drain the corn and allow to steam-dry for a few seconds. Take a spoonful of the satay sauce and rub it all over the outside of the corn.

Serve a corn on the cob alongside a piece of griddled chicken with the salad leaves on the side.

Per serving 394 cals | 38g protein | 21g fat (4g saturates) | 12g carbs (5g total sugars) | 4g fibre

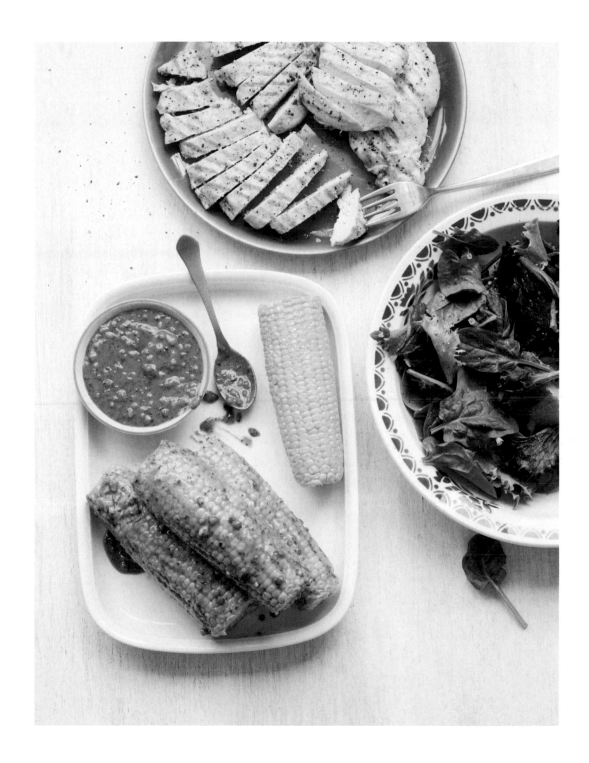

Get Ahead

FREEZER MAGIC

BEEF, VEGETABLE AND PEARL BARLEY STEW

This warming stew is great for weekends when you've got time to spend on cooking. If you make the full amount, you can put leftovers in the freezer so you'll never be short of a super tasty lunch or dinner. It contains wholesome pearl barley (you'll find it in supermarkets near the pasta or rice), which will fill you up so there's absolutely no excuse for any stodgy potatoes or dumplings on the side.

Makes 6 portions

1 tbsp olive oil

1 onion, diced

2 sticks of celery, diced

1 large carrot, peeled and diced

1 leek, halved and cut into 1 cm slices

2 tbsp brown rice flour

1kg lean stewing steak

1 small celeriac, peeled and cut into chunks

1.5 litres fresh vegetable or beef stock

4 fresh thyme sprigs

2 bay leaves

150g pearl barley

Sea salt and freshly ground black pepper

Preheat the oven to 170°C/Fan 150°C/Gas 3. Heat the oil in a large casserole pot over a medium-high heat. Add the onion, celery, carrot and leek, and sweat gently for 10 minutes. Stir frequently to make sure nothing sticks – you just want everything to soften.

Sprinkle the rice flour over the stewing steak, add to the pot and cook for 5 minutes until it is sealed on all sides. Add the celeriac chunks and the vegetable stock. This should cover everything in the pot – if not, just top it up with a little water. Add the sprigs of thyme and the bay leaves. Turn off the heat.

Put the lid on the casserole pot and pop it into the oven for 1 hour.

After the hour is up, rinse the pearl barley in a sieve under cold running water and then add to the pot. Replace the lid and return it to the oven for another 45 minutes. Stir once halfway through this time.

Remove the lid and return the pot to the oven for another 15–30 minutes, until the meat just falls apart.

Remove the sprigs of thyme and the bay leaves, and season to taste. Divide into six portions and enjoy!

Per serving 397 cals | 43g protein | 10g fat (3g saturates) | 32g carbs (7g total sugars) | 5g fibre

LAMB KOFTE WITH LETTUCE WRAPS

Think of this as a healthy kebab! Koftes are a protein powerhouse, and the spiced meat really hits the spot. If you've got the time to let the red onions sit and pickle, it's totally worth doing – they are very simple to do, but they add an amazing zingy crunch to the finished kofte wraps.

Makes 8 portions

For the kofte:

1kg lamb mince
1 tbsp dried mint
2 tsp ground cumin
1 tsp ground cinnamon
½ tsp ground nutmeg
20g fresh flat-leaf parsley, roughly chopped
Freshly ground black pepper, to taste

For the quick pickled onions:

2 red onions, thinly sliced
1 tsp salt
1 tsp black peppercorns
100ml red wine vinegar

Per person, per serving:

2 cos lettuce leaves
20g 0% fat Greek yoghurt
Handful of fresh mint leaves
Chilli flakes

Put all the ingredients for the kofte in a large mixing bowl and use your hands to mix and knead everything together. Divide the mixture into 16 balls (about 65g each) and roll them into sausage shapes 10cm long.

If you want to freeze them, now is the perfect time. Tear up some non-stick baking paper into pieces as long as the kofte and twice as wide. Lay each kofte on a piece of paper. Place them (with the paper) in an airtight container, using the paper to stop them touching one another. This will make it easier when you take them out of the freezer later on.

If you are eating them straight away, push a metal skewer gently through the middle of each kofte. Give the meat mix a little squeeze to bond it to the skewer. Allow two kofte per person. Place the skewers in the fridge to firm up for 30 minutes before cooking

Meanwhile, make the quick pickled onions. Boil a kettle of water and place the sliced red onions in a heat-proof bowl. Sprinkle over the salt and add the peppercorns. Add the red wine vinegar and enough boiling water to cover the onions. Leave to one side to pickle for a minimum of 15 minutes. They will keep in the fridge for a week or two.

Once you are ready to eat, heat a large frying pan or griddle – you shouldn't need to add any oil, as the fat in the lamb will quickly start to ooze out. Add the kofte (in batches, if needed) and cook for 8–10 minutes, turning every couple of minutes to make sure they cook evenly and get a deep brown colour all over. Take a lettuce leaf, slide off a kofte and place it on the leaf. Top with a dollop of Greek yoghurt, some pickled red onion, some fresh mint leaves and a sprinkle of chilli flakes.

Per serving 276 cals | 27g protein | 17g fat (8g saturates) | 4g carbs (3g total sugars) | 1g fibre

PASTA-FREE LASAGNE

I don't eat pasta, but that doesn't mean I don't still want to enjoy a lovely lasagne, and this one tastes unbelievable. Its layers are made up of courgette and aubergine slices, and the Bolognese sauce includes hearty Puy lentils, which means less meat is needed. If you're vegetarian you can omit the beef completely and and either use Quorn or just double the amount of lentils.

Makes 6 portions

3 tbsp olive oil

1 red onion, diced

2 sticks of celery, diced

1 large carrot, peeled and diced

3 garlic cloves, finely grated

1 tbsp tomato purée

250g beef mince, 5% fat

250g pre-cooked Puy lentils

1 tbsp dried oregano

1 tsp ground nutmeg

2 x 400g tins chopped tomatoes

2 courgettes, cut lengthways into 3mm slices

2 aubergines, cut into 3mm rounds

30g butter

30g brown rice flour

450ml skimmed milk

Preheat the oven to 180°C/Fan 160°C/Gas 4.

Heat one tablespoon of the olive oil in a large saucepan over a medium-high heat. Add the onion, celery and carrot. Allow them to cook gently over a medium heat for 6–7 minutes, so they really start to soften and turn golden brown. Add the garlic and cook for 30 seconds until it becomes aromatic.

Add the tomato purée and cook for 1 minute before adding the beef mince. Increase the heat and cook until the meat is no longer pink but browned all over, stirring regularly.

Add the lentils and stir well to incorporate, along with the oregano and half the nutmeg.

Stir in the chopped tomatoes and bring everything up to boiling point. Reduce the heat and cook at a gentle simmer for around 30 minutes, stirring occasionally, until it starts to thicken.

While the Bolognese sauce is cooking away, you can prepare the courgettes and aubergines. Heat a griddle pan and when it's really hot, lightly brush one side of the courgette slices and one side of the aubergine rounds with a little of the remaining oil. Place them on the griddle pan, oiled side down. Cook for around 90 seconds, then

cont ...

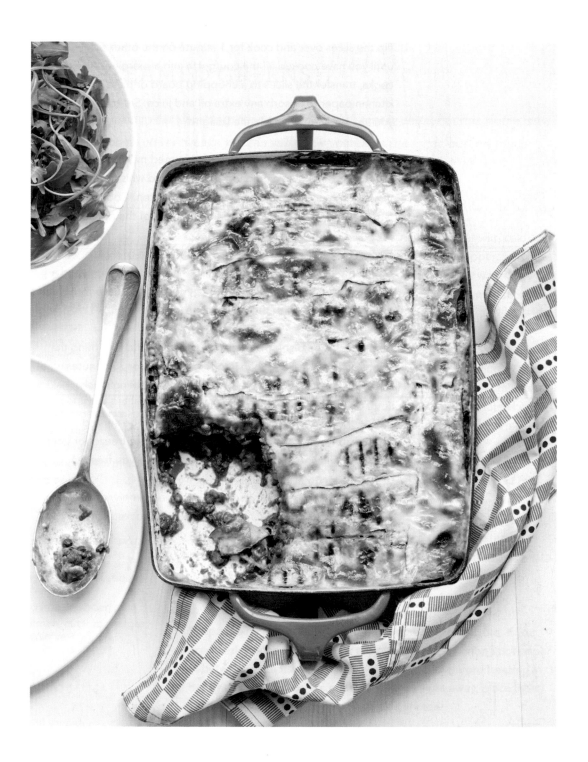

PRAWN CHILLI PANCAKES
AND CUCUMBER SALAD

I love, love, love these, and so does everyone I've ever made them for. Whenever I've taken them on set for lunch I've had to pack extra because everyone wants to try them. The cucumber salad is really refreshing on the side.

Serves 4
Makes 8 pancakes
(2 per serving)

2 garlic cloves, finely grated

3cm piece of ginger,
    peeled and grated

1 stalk of lemongrass,
    outer leaves removed
    and finely chopped

1 banana shallot,
    finely chopped

2 red chillis, finely chopped

10g fresh coriander,
    roughly chopped

300g raw prawns,
    roughly chopped

2 medium eggs

1 tbsp olive oil

For the cucumber salad
(for 2 servings):

1 cucumber

2 spring onions, sliced

1 tsp low-salt soy sauce

1 tsp toasted sesame oil

Pinch of salt

1 tsp chilli flakes (optional),
    to garnish

Place the garlic, ginger, lemongrass, banana shallot, chilli and coriander in a food processor and blitz into a rough paste. Add the prawns, then crack in the eggs and carry on blitzing until everything has made a thick paste. Set to one side.

Cut the cucumber in half and then into chunks. Place them in a mixing bowl with a pinch of salt. Use the end of a rolling pin to bash the pieces and soften them. Add the spring onions, soy sauce and sesame oil. Mix well and then set aside while you cook the pancakes.

Heat the olive oil in a non-stick frying pan over a medium-high heat. Once the oil is hot, swoosh it round the pan to coat the base. Place spoonfuls of the prawn mixture in the frying pan, shaping them with the spoon to make round, even pancakes about 1cm thick. You may need to do this in a couple of batches. Cook each side for 3–4 minutes, pressing down with a spatula occasionally to help them keep their shape. This also helps remove any excess water from inside the pancakes while they're cooking (which might make them soggy when you're eating them). Once they are done, remove from the pan and keep warm until you have made them all.

If you'd like to freeze some pancakes, allow them to fully cool before placing some non-stick baking paper between them and wrapping them in cling film. You can then freeze them in handy batches.

Serve the prawn chilli pancakes alongside the cucumber salad. Garnish with chilli flakes for an extra kick, if desired.

Per serving (2 pancakes, including salad) 136 cals | 17g protein | 7g fat (1g saturates) | 1g carbs (1g total sugars) | 1g fibre

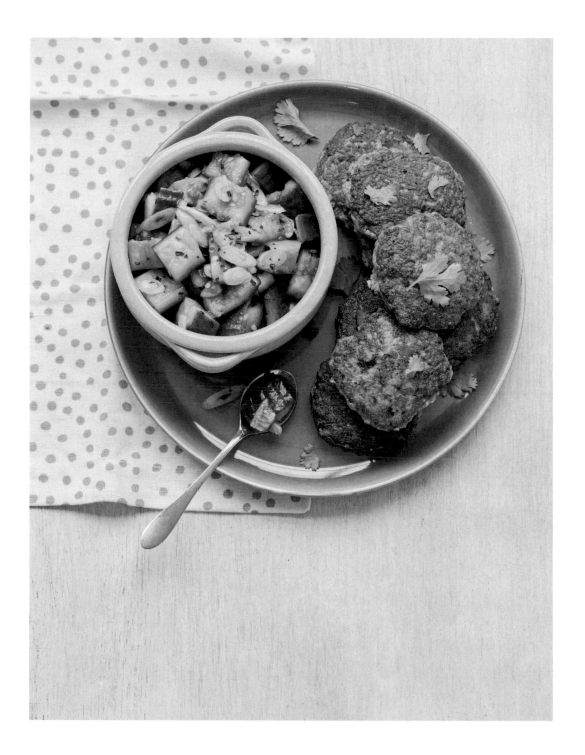

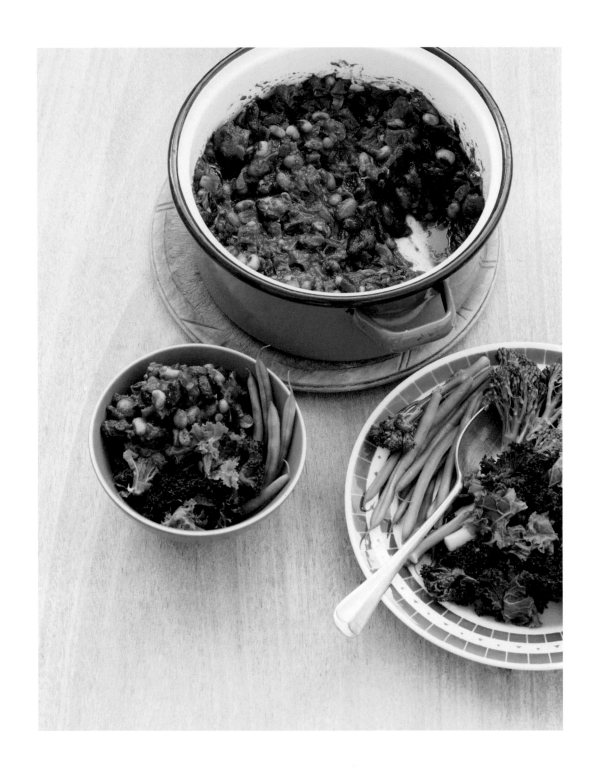

SPICY BEAN CHILLI

Don't be freaked out by the espresso shot in this spice sensation. It works, trust me! You can simply make up a shot with some instant espresso powder if you don't have a fancy machine. Gone are the days when I used to pile my chilli on to a big buttery baked potato. Now I have it on a hearty heap of steamed greens, or sometimes just on its own.

Makes 4–6 portions

1 tsp olive oil

1 red onion, diced

1 green chilli, chopped

2 garlic cloves, finely grated

1 tbsp tomato purée

1 x 400g tin kidney beans, drained

1 x 400g tin borlotti beans, drained

1 x 400g tin black-eyed beans, drained

1 tbsp chilli flakes

1 tbsp dried oregano

1 tsp ground cinnamon

2 x 400g tins chopped tomatoes

1 espresso shot

Heat the olive oil in a large casserole pot over a medium-high heat. Add the onion and chilli. Cook for 5 minutes until the onion has started to soften and turn golden brown. Add the garlic and cook for another 30 seconds.

Add the tomato purée and cook for 30 seconds, then add all the beans and mix well. Sprinkle over the chilli flakes, oregano and cinnamon, and stir to incorporate. Add the chopped tomatoes and coffee.

Mix everything together and bring up to the boil. Reduce the heat and simmer gently, stirring occasionally, for around 20–25 minutes, until the chilli has reduced and thickened up.

This is wonderful served on top of a heap of steamed greens (sweetheart cabbage, Savoy cabbage, cavolo nero, green beans, etc.), in which case it will feed six people. But if you just want a bowl of chilli, it will feed four.

Any leftovers should be allowed to cool down to room temperature before being divided into portions and stored in the fridge or freezer for later use.

Per serving (for 6 servings) 185 cals | 11g protein | 2g fat (0g saturates) | 27g carbs (8g total sugars) | 10g fibre

BUTTERNUT SQUASH AND GOAT'S CHEESE FILO TART

Filo is the only kind of pastry I eat because it's quite a lot healthier than other types. It adds a lovely crisp crunch to the softer ingredients in this yummy tart. This can easily be cut up into small portions and taken in slices for lunch, or even served as canapés!

Makes 6 portions

400g butternut squash, peeled and cut into 1cm cubes

1 tsp olive oil

1 small onion, diced

2 garlic cloves, finely grated

10 sage leaves, roughly chopped

Knob of butter

125g filo pastry

5 large eggs

A pinch of freshly ground nutmeg

120g soft goat's cheese

Sea salt and freshly ground black pepper

Preheat the oven to 190°C/Fan 170°C/Gas 5.

Fill a saucepan with 5cm of water and bring to the boil with a steamer basket and lid on top. Once the water is boiling, add the butternut squash to the steamer basket. Steam the squash for 10–12 minutes until tender all the way through, but not soft, then remove from the heat and allow the squash to steam-dry.

While the squash steams, heat the oil in a frying pan over a medium-high heat and add the onion. Cook for 5 minutes to soften before adding the garlic and sage. Add the squash and continue to cook for another minute, then remove from the heat and allow to cool a little.

To make the tart case, take a 23cm loose-bottomed tart tin and use the knob of butter to very lightly grease the base and sides of the tin so the pastry won't stick. Take a sheet of pastry and lay it in the tin, pressing it very carefully into the crease round the base. Leave some of the pastry hanging over the edge so you have a nice crispy crust.

Separate one of the eggs; place the white in a small cup and the yolk in a large jug. Brush the pastry with a little egg white and then layer on another sheet of pastry. Repeat until you have used all the pastry. Make sure there are no holes in the base and that you have at least four good layers on the base.

cont . . .

Per serving 239 cals | 13g protein | 12g fat (6g saturates) | 18g carbs (4g total sugars) | 2g fibre

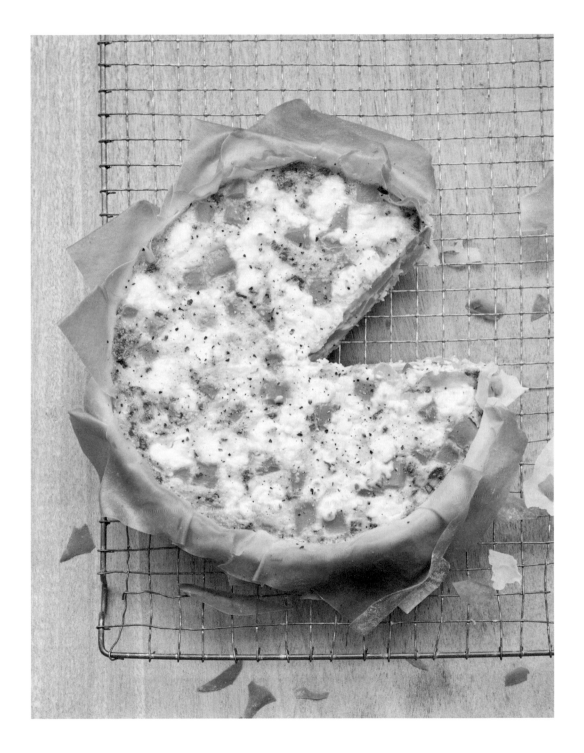

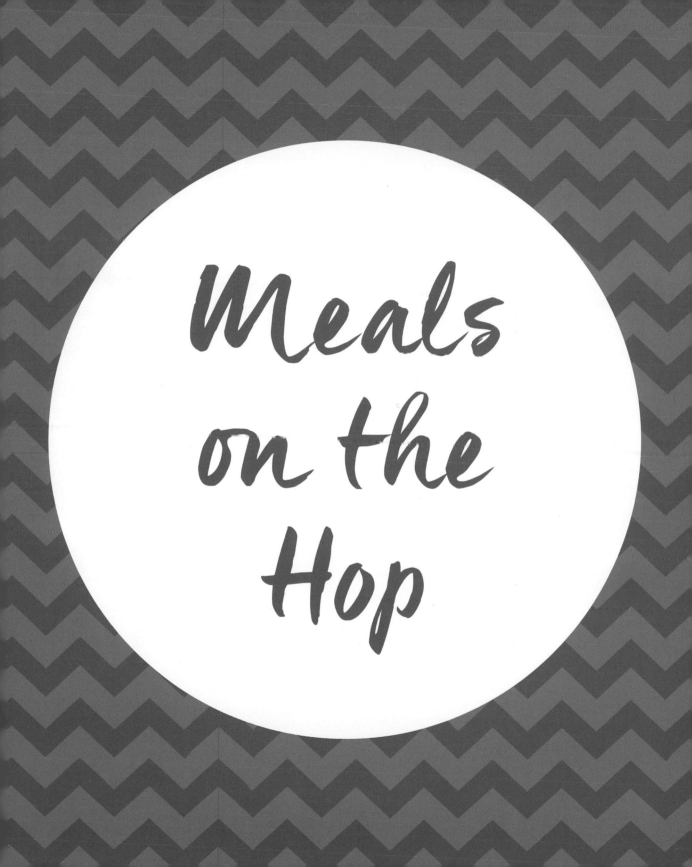

Meals
on the
Hop

OVERNIGHT CHIA OATS
WITH BERRIES

Lots of people think chia seeds are faffy and a bit of a fad, but they're honestly dead easy and so, so good for you, as they're full of fibre and protein. You can get them in supermarkets now, but also in health food shops, as well as online. If you can't find them, this recipe can just be made without.

Serves 1

30g rolled oats

2 tbsp chia seeds

180ml oat milk/cashew milk/almond milk/coconut milk

30g frozen berries (raspberries, strawberries, blackberries, redcurrants)

This is a recipe where you can simply stick everything in a jar or airtight container that fits the ingredients snugly, and mix together well. Give the jar a good shake to mix, then pop it into the fridge the night before you need it.

Lisa's tip: A great trick is to make a batch of the dry ingredients in a big jar, and then just decant a serving when you want. All you need do is add the milk and berries each evening. You can just grab it in the morning and go!

Per serving 340 cals | 11g protein | 14g fat (2g saturates) | 36g carbs (7g total sugars) | 15g fibre

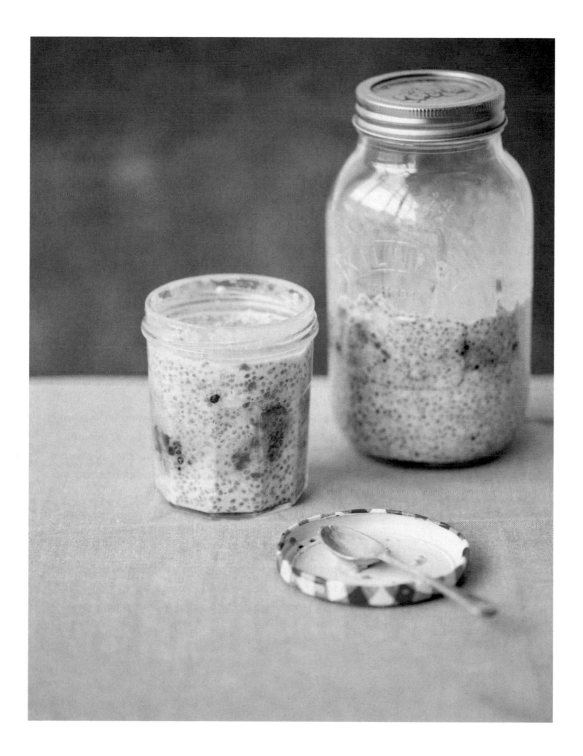

SPINACH, BROCCOLI, KIWI AND GREEK YOGHURT SMOOTHIE

This may sound like quite a weird concoction but the combination of sweet and savoury together really works. Also, if your tummy ever feels a bit upset, the ginger in this will help to settle things down.

Serves 1

60g frozen spinach
75g frozen broccoli
1 kiwi, peeled and
   roughly chopped
1cm ginger, peeled
and finely chopped
60g 0% fat Greek yoghurt
180–220ml cold water

Place all the ingredients in a blender and run on high until everything is super smooth. This will take 1–2 minutes, depending on how powerful your blender is. Add a little more water if you prefer a looser mix.

The beauty of using frozen vegetables is that they make a deliciously cold frozen smoothie. This makes for a smoother mix than using fresh raw vegetables.

Per serving 117 cals | 12g protein | 1g fat (0g saturates) | 12g carbs (11g total sugars) | 6g fibre

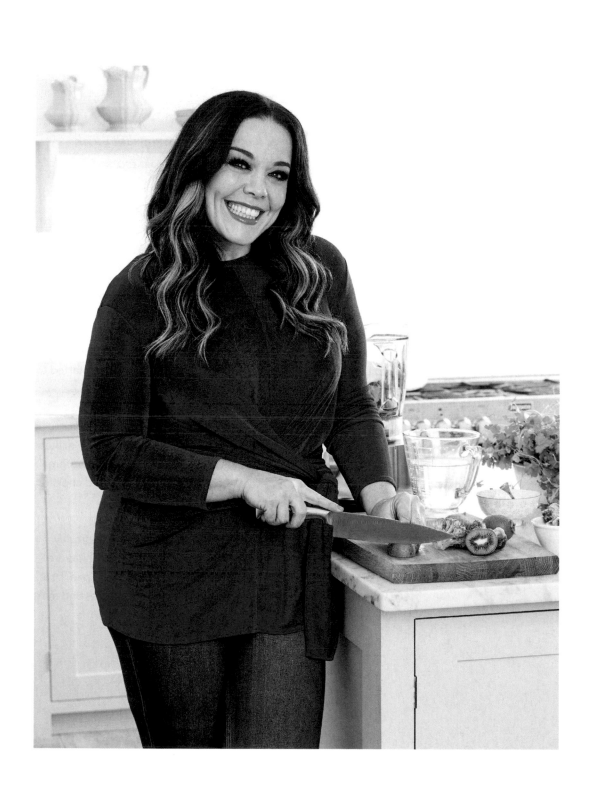

SKINNY OMELETTE WRAPS

I am obsessed with eggs, so I love finding new ways to use them in recipes. As you know, I don't eat bread or regular wheat wraps, so I often use omelettes as wraps instead. These are a brilliant Sunday brunch option if you've had a bit of a lie in. Once you have this trick up your sleeve, you can vary the fillings to whatever you prefer.

Serves 2
(Makes 2 wraps)

1 tbsp olive oil
2 medium eggs, beaten
1 tbsp chopped dill
1 tbsp 0% fat Greek
  yoghurt
Half an avocado, sliced
20g rocket leaves
50g smoked salmon
Freshly ground black
  pepper

Heat half the oil in a small frying pan over a medium-high heat, then add half the beaten eggs and tip the pan around to make sure you cover the whole base in a thin, even layer. Sprinkle over half the dill. Cook for around 1½ minutes, until the top has stopped looking wet. Then flip the omelette and cook for another 30 seconds on the other side. Slide the omelette out on to a plate and repeat to make the other wrap.

Once you have both your wraps, dot half the Greek yoghurt over each. Divide the avocado, rocket and smoked salmon between them. Season with a little black pepper and then roll them up. These wraps are brilliant to take with you in the morning, as they are delicious hot or cold.

Per serving 206 cals | 9g protein | 18g fat (5g saturates) | 2g carbs (2g total sugars) | 2g fibre

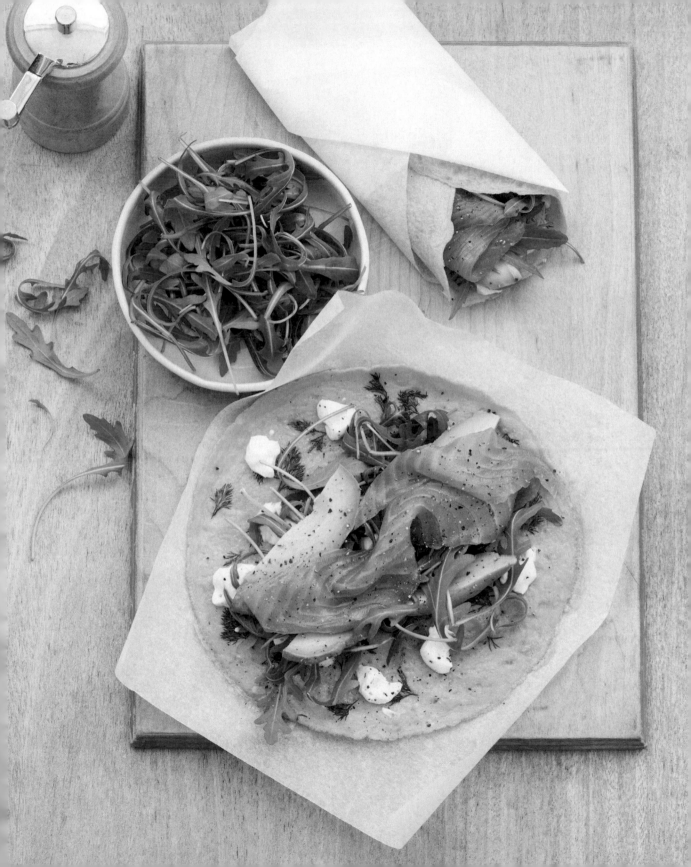

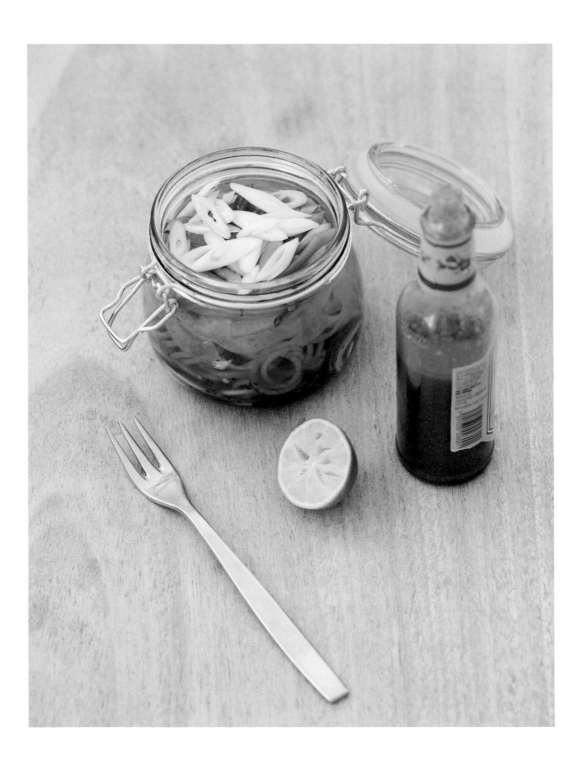

HOT AND SOUR VEGGIE NOODLE SOUP

Forget Pot Noodles, this is your new on-the-go lunch solution! A bit of speedy prep in the morning or the night before – for which you need a cheap spiralizer (see page 142 – mine has changed my life!) – then stick the jar in your bag as you run out the door. When you're ready for lunch, all you need is a kettle . . . and hey presto!

Serves 1

1 chicken or vegetable stock pot
1 tsp chilli flakes
1 tsp hot sauce (Tabasco/ Cholula, etc.)
1 courgette, spiralized
1 medium carrot, spiralized
1 yellow pepper, deseeded and spiralized
40g sugar snap peas, halved lengthways
2 spring onions, thinly sliced
320ml boiling water
Juice of half a lime

Put the stock pot, chilli flakes and hot sauce in the bottom of a jar (or airtight container), and carefully layer up the courgette, carrot and pepper noodles. Top with the sugar snap peas and spring onions. This is all you need to do before popping the lid on and keeping it in the fridge until you are ready.

When you are ready to eat, boil a kettle and add the hot water to the jar. Allow the vegetables to soften in the hot water for 5–10 minutes (depending on how crunchy you like them) before gently shaking or stirring the contents to make a broth from the stock pot.

Squeeze the lime juice over the top and tuck in. Hot, sour, spicy and crunchy lunch on the go!

Per serving 134 cals | 6g protein | 3g fat (0g saturates) | 17g carbs (16g total sugars) | 9g fibre

BEETROOT, CRANBERRY AND POMEGRANATE SALAD
WITH LIME AND BALSAMIC DRESSING

The days of salads just being made up of lettuce and cucumber are over! You will want to savour every mouthful of this one. Pomegranate molasses is a thick dark sauce a bit like a balsamic vinegar, but sweeter and sharper. If you don't have any, just leave it out and add the juice from the rest of the lime instead.

Serves 1

50g mixed green
    salad leaves
150g cooked beetroot,
    quartered
30g dried cranberries
30g pomegranate seeds
20g toasted walnuts
15g toasted pumpkin
    seeds

For the dressing:

Juice of half a lime
1 tsp pomegranate
    molasses
1 tbsp balsamic vinegar
Freshly ground black
    pepper

To make this salad to go, get yourself a big jar or airtight container. Layer the leaves in the base, topped with the beetroot, cranberries and pomegranate seeds. Then add the walnuts and pumpkin seeds.

In a little pot mix together the lime juice, pomegranate molasses and balsamic vinegar and as much black pepper as you like.

Add the dressing to the salad ingredients and give it a little shake to coat everything. Delicious!

Lisa's tip: You could add the dressing to the salad straight away, but if you're taking it with you for later in the day, the leaves will stay crunchier if you add it just before you eat.

Per serving 462 cals | 12g protein | 22g fat (3g saturates) | 50g carbs (40g total sugars) | 10g fibre

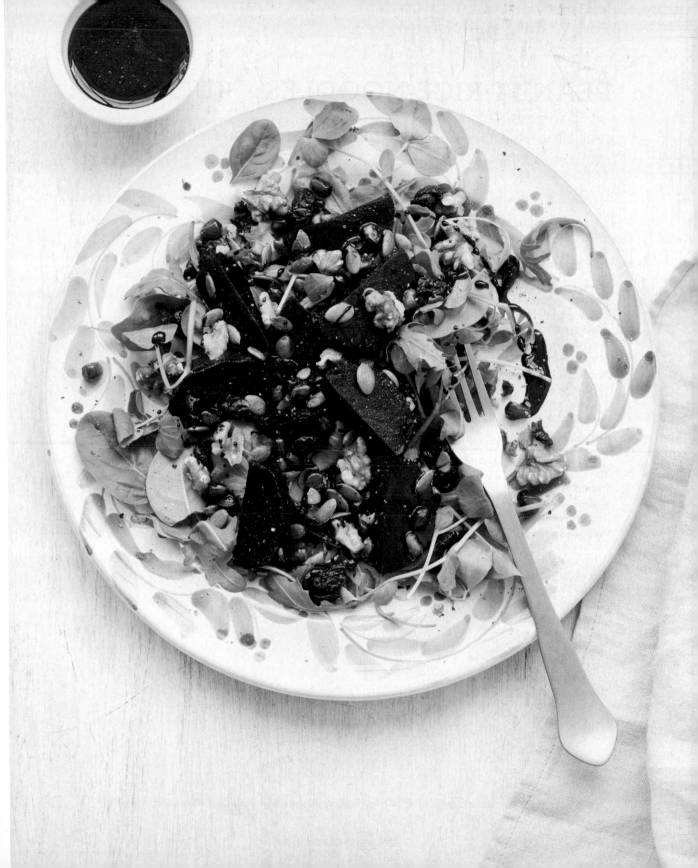

VEGGIE SUSHI
WITH QUINOA

I still can't believe I make my own sushi, but with all the ingredients so readily available in supermarkets now I'd be crazy not to. Plus, it looks super impressive. If you're not usually a sushi fan, rest assured there's no raw fish in sight here, it's all vegetables.

Serves 2

400g pre-cooked quinoa
2 tsp rice wine vinegar
4 nori seaweed sheets
1 tbsp 0% fat Greek yoghurt
1 tsp wasabi paste (optional)
1 avocado, thinly sliced
1 carrot, peeled and cut into matchsticks
Half a cucumber, peeled, deseeded and cut into matchsticks

Weigh out the quinoa into a saucepan and add double the amount of cold water. Bring the water to the boil and then simmer with the lid on for 12–14 minutes (or according to the packet instructions).

Drain the quinoa, then sprinkle over the rice wine vinegar. Stir to mix, then allow to cool and steam-dry for a few minutes.

Once the quinoa is cool, take a sushi rolling mat and lay a sheet of nori on it. Take a quarter of the quinoa and gently spread it all over the nori, leaving a 2cm gap on the side closest to you and the side furthest from you. Gently press down on the filling with the back of a spoon to encourage it to stick together and to flatten it out.

Mix the yoghurt and wasabi, if using, together. Leaving a 2cm gap of quinoa at the front of the nori, spread a stripe about 3cm wide across the width of the quinoa. Add a quarter of the avocado slices on top of that, followed by a quarter of the carrot and cucumber.

Then very gently use the sushi mat to help you start to roll the sushi up. Go slowly, making sure you keep it as tight as possible, until it is almost all rolled. Wet your finger in a little water and gently pat it on the side of the nori furthest from you. Keep rolling until the damp nori connects with the roll, as this will seal it and keep its shape.

Cut each roll into five pieces. This will keep in the fridge overnight, but the nori will soften.

Per serving 595 cals | 21g protein | 24g fat (3g saturates) | 64g carbs (9g total sugars) | 20g fibre

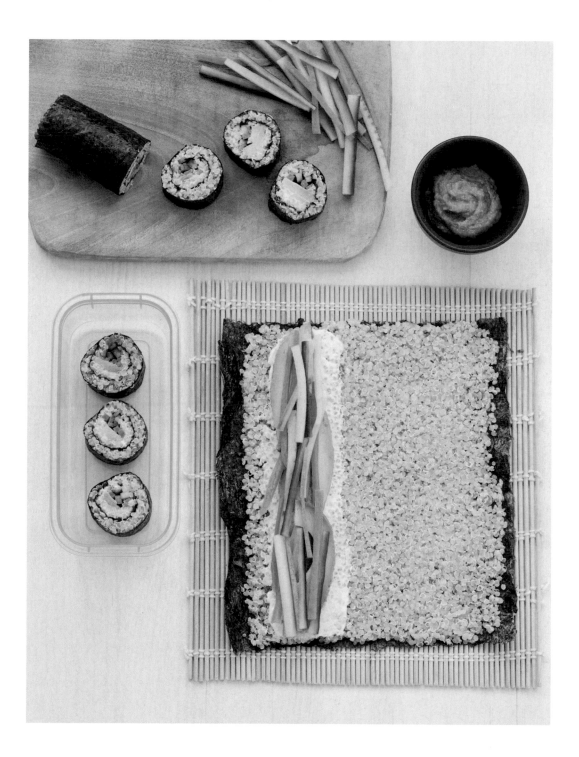

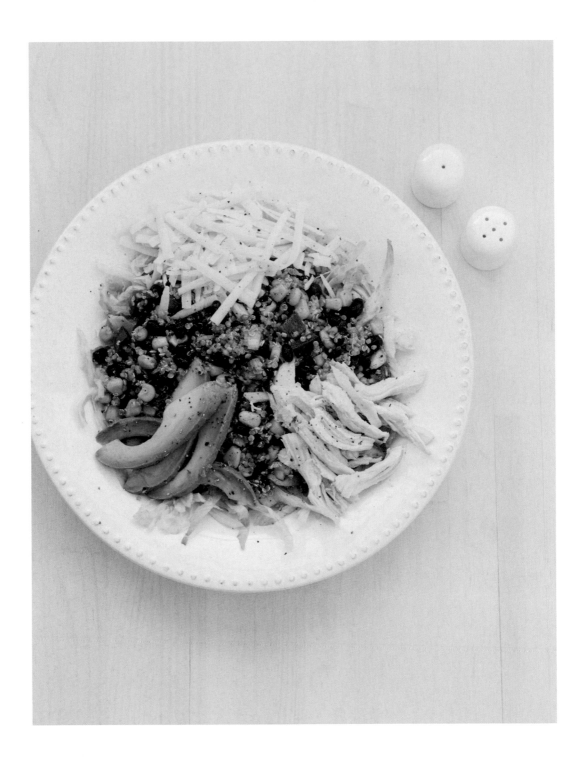

DECONSTRUCTED BURRITO BOWL

Not only does this taste so good – like fireworks are going off in your mouth – it also looks amazing. Think burritos, but without the heavy distractions of rice or wraps. It's a great recipe for whipping up with leftover chicken and quinoa.

Makes 4 portions

250g pre-cooked quinoa

1 x 400g tin black beans, drained and rinsed

1 x 185g tin sweetcorn, drained

1 red pepper, deseeded and diced

1 banana shallot, finely diced

1 tsp sweet smoked paprika

½ tsp cumin

½ tsp garlic powder

Juice of 1 lime

1 tbsp olive oil

Per person, to serve:

50g iceberg lettuce, shredded

20g low-fat Cheddar cheese, grated

Quarter of an avocado, sliced

75g cooked chicken, shredded

Sea salt and freshly ground black pepper

Put the pre-cooked quinoa into a mixing bowl along with the black beans, sweetcorn, red pepper and banana shallot.

Add the spices, garlic, lime juice and olive oil and mix everything together until it is all evenly coated. This will keep in the fridge for 3–4 days.

For each serving, place the iceberg lettuce in the base of a bowl/ jar or airtight container. Top with some of the quinoa mix, Cheddar, avocado and shredded chicken.

Add a little extra seasoning if you like. Pop the lid on, and you're good to go.

Per serving 507 cals | 40g protein | 19g fat (5g saturates) | 37g carbs (7g total sugars) | 11g fibre

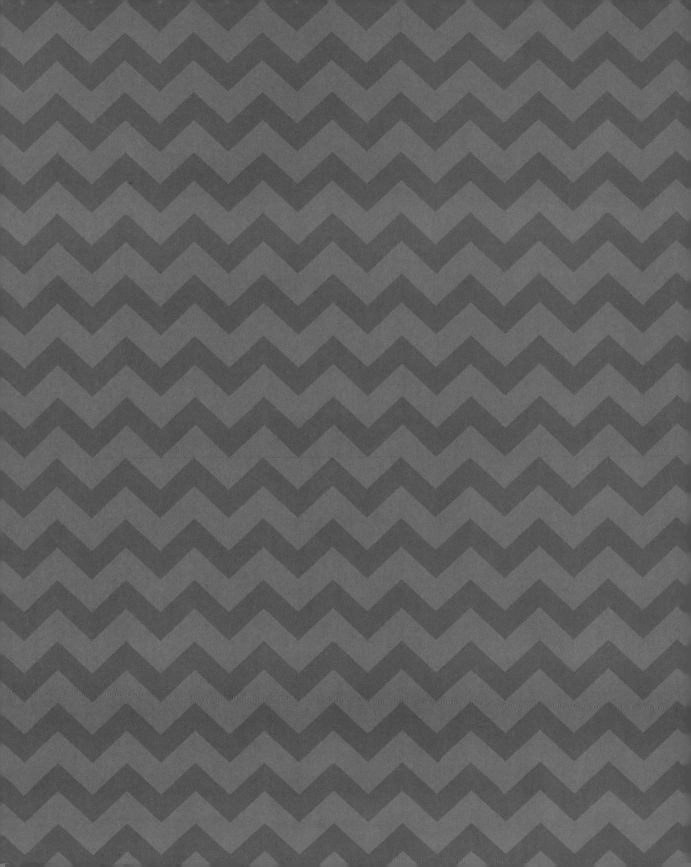

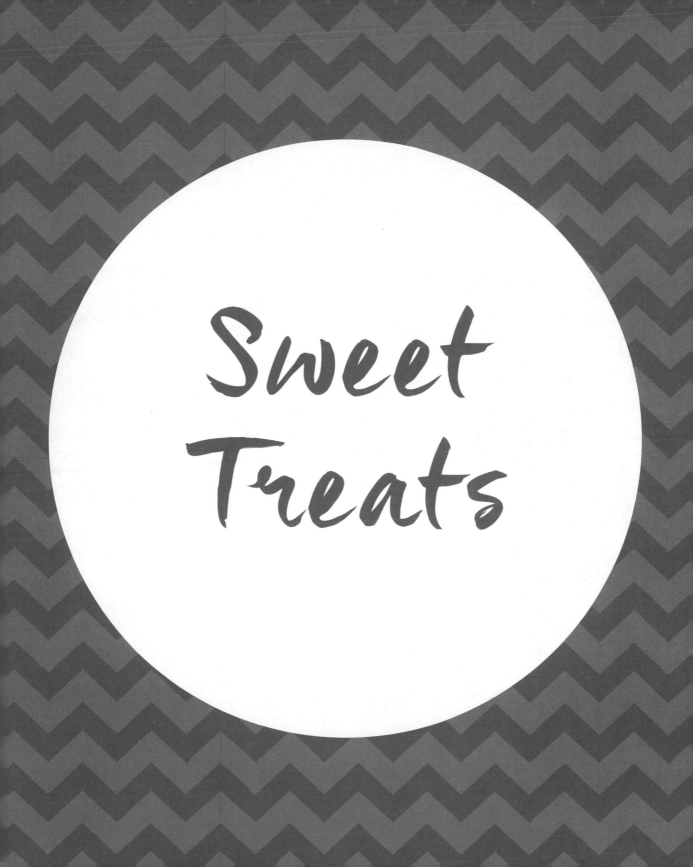

Sweet
Treats

RASPBERRY SORBET

Who knew it was so easy to make sorbet? If you've got a tub of this in your freezer you're always set if you fancy a sweet treat.

Serves 6

500g frozen raspberries, thawed
50ml runny honey
Juice of 1 lemon

Blitz everything together in a food processor until it is all broken down into a smooth purée. Pass it through a sieve, to remove all the seeds, straight into a 1-litre freezer-proof tub with a lid.

Place the tub in the freezer for about 3 hours (until it is 80 per cent frozen), then remove and blitz the sorbet again. Put it back into the tub and freeze overnight.

Lisa's tip: Using frozen fruit is ideal for this, as you can make it out of season, all year round – plus frozen berries are much friendlier on the purse.

Per serving 53 cals | 1g protein | 0g fat (0g saturates) | 10g carbs (10g total sugars) | 3g fibre

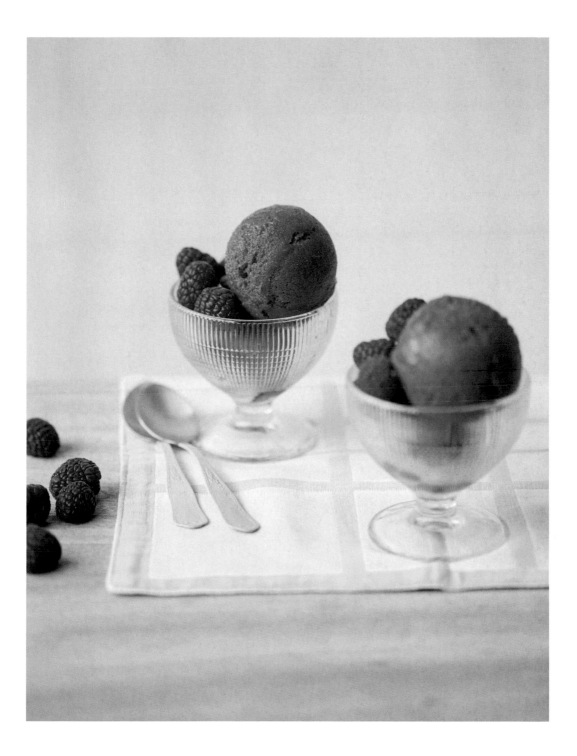

FRUIT LOLLIES

I've made these often, and they're so easy that I genuinely think I could whip them up with my eyes closed! Just two or three ingredients = the most amazing flavours. Not surprisingly, my nephews love the raspberry ones and the mango ones. The watermelon and ginger lollies are a bit more grown-up, but the kids can't have all the fun, right?

Serves 4

For the raspberry and coconut frozen yoghurt lollies:

120g raspberries
150g low-fat coconut yoghurt
100ml coconut water

For the mango and coconut lollies:

150g ripe mango, diced
200ml coconut water

For the watermelon and ginger lollies:

300g watermelon, roughly chopped and seeds removed
5g ginger, peeled

To make the raspberry and coconut frozen yoghurt lollies, place all the ingredients in a jug and stir to mix. Using the end of a rolling pin, gently break up the raspberries a little to release the juices. Give the jug another gentle stir to swirl the berries through the yoghurt. Fill four 65ml lolly moulds to just below the rim and pop the sticks in. Place in the freezer overnight, and enjoy the next day.

To make the mango and coconut lollies, place the mango and coconut water in a jug and use a stick blender to blitz until it is very smooth. Pour into four 65ml lolly moulds until just below the rim. Pop the sticks in, and freeze overnight.

To make the watermelon and ginger lollies, place the watermelon and ginger in a jug and use a stick blender to blitz until it is very smooth. Pour into four 65ml lolly moulds until just below the rim. Pop the sticks in, and freeze overnight.

Per serving (raspberry) 63 cals | 1g protein | 5g fat (4g saturates) | 3g carbs (3g total sugars) | 1g fibre
Per serving (mango) 34 cals | 0g protein | 0g fat (0g saturates) | 8g carbs (7g total sugars) | 1g fibre
Per serving (watermelon) 24 cals | 0g protein | 0g fat (0g saturates) | 5g carbs (5g total sugars) | 0g fibre

FRUIT JELLY

Forget kids' parties, it's time to reclaim the jelly! This one looks good, tastes good and even provides some of your five a day!

Makes 1 large jelly
(Feeds 6 people)

1 x sachet sugar-free orange jelly crystals

285ml boiling water

285ml cold water

2 small oranges, segmented

30g pomegranate seeds

Place the jelly crystals in a pudding basin or jelly mould and add boiling water, according to the packet instructions. Stir until the crystals have all dissolved. Add the cold water and allow to cool down to room temperature before adding the fruit to the jelly.

Pop the jelly into the fridge to set overnight.

Lisa's tip: There is a whole range of sugar-free, low-calorie jellies available. Try experimenting with a raspberry jelly and a handful of fresh red berries; or a blackcurrant jelly with a handful of blackberries to keep it interesting.

Per serving 19 cals | 1g protein | 0g fat (0g saturates) | 4g carbs (3g total sugars) | 1g fibre

ZESTY ZERO COCKTAIL

If you're having the girls round in summer, they'll be well impressed with this. It's also a great way to perk up water if you're trying to make yourself drink more and keep well hydrated.

Serves 1

Juice of 1 lime
5 raspberries
1 orange slice
1 lemon slice
300ml sparkling water
Ice cubes, to serve
Fresh mint leaves, to serve

Put the lime juice, raspberries and orange and lemon slices into a large tumbler. Fill the tumbler with sparkling water.

Add a few ice cubes. Top with mint leaves and enjoy!

Per serving 2 cals | 0g protein | 0g fat (0g saturates) | <1g carbs (<1g total sugars) | 0g fibre

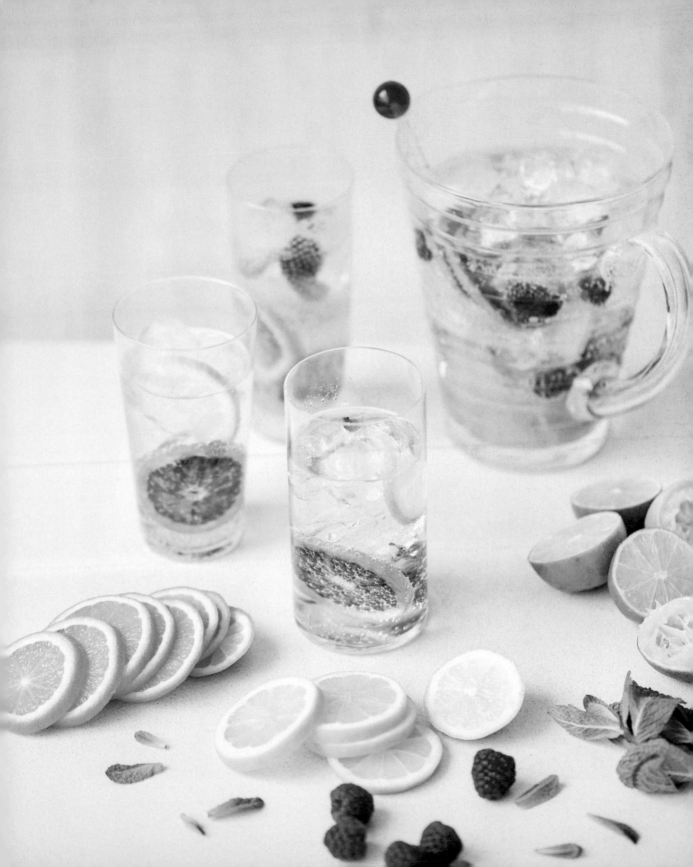

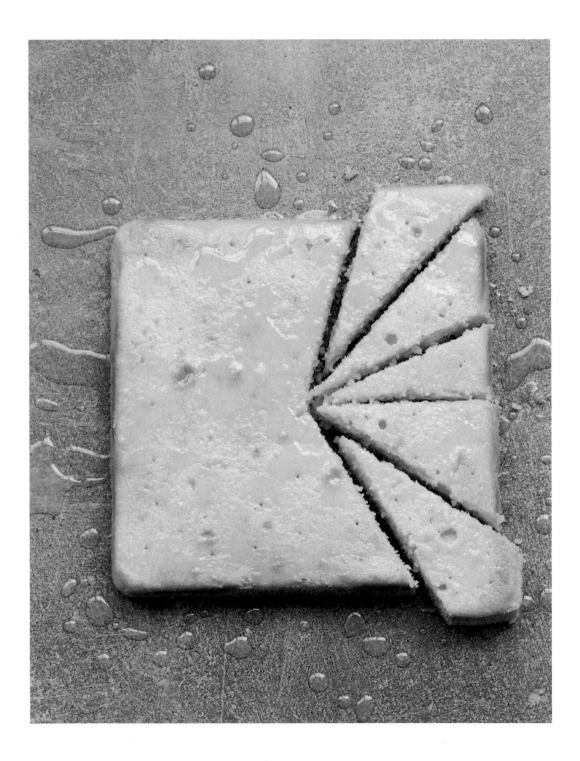

LEMON DRIZZLE TRAY BAKE

This is one of my dearest recipes of all time because it always reminds me of my amazing mum. It was one of her absolute favourites and it makes me think of the incredible times we had together. Even though I've created a healthier version of the old classic, it still contains sugar, so is best kept as an end-of-diet treat.

Makes 12–16 portions

150g low-fat spread
100g caster sugar
3 medium eggs, beaten
100g plain flour
100g ground almonds
1 tsp baking powder
3 tbsp almond milk
Juice and zest of 2 lemons

For the drizzle:

100g icing sugar
Juice of 1½ lemons

Preheat the oven to 180°C/Fan 160°C/Gas 4. Line a 20cm square cake tin with non-stick baking paper.

Beat the low-fat spread and sugar together in a mixing bowl with an electric whisk until pale and fluffy. Add the eggs, plain flour, ground almonds and baking powder and beat again until everything is incorporated. Add the milk and the zest of both lemons (reserving the juice for the drizzle) and gently stir in.

Pour the cake batter into the lined baking tin, gently spread out and place the tin in the oven for 20–22 minutes.

While the cake is baking, make the drizzle by dissolving the icing sugar in the juice from one and a half of the zested lemons in a small saucepan. Place on a very low heat and warm it very gently to just help the sugar dissolve, then set to one side until you need it.

The cake is done when it has risen and turned a light golden brown around the edges. A cocktail stick or skewer inserted into the middle should come out clean. Remove the cake from the oven and use the cocktail stick or skewer to make holes all over the top of the cake. Pour the drizzle over the cake, making sure everything gets a good soaking. Allow to sit and absorb for 15 minutes.

Carefully use the baking paper to lift the cake out of the tin. Remove the baking paper and place the cake on to a wire rack to cool fully.

Per serving (for 16): 158 cals | 3g protein | 8g fat (1g saturates) | 18g carbs (13g total sugars) | 1g fibre

CHOCOLATE BANANA ICE CREAM

Obviously this isn't something you should be eating on a daily basis, but it makes a brilliant, healthy dessert the whole family will be happy to tuck into. It's a handy way to use up over-ripe bananas too.

Serves 6

450g ripe bananas
2–3 tbsp unsweetened cocoa powder (according to taste)

Start by cutting the bananas into ½cm-thick slices. Lay them out on a tray or baking sheet that will fit into your freezer – you might need more than one. Freeze for an hour, then remove and pop the slices into a food processor along with the cocoa powder. You want the banana to be about 80 per cent frozen so it will still blend easily.

Blitz the banana and cocoa together to make instant ice cream. If it gets a bit runny while you're blitzing it, all you need to do is pop it back into the freezer in a freezer-proof container to firm up – and this is also how you can store any leftovers.

Once frozen, take the ice cream out of the freezer 10 minutes before serving so it can start to soften and be scoopable!

Per serving 82 cals | 2g protein | 1g fat (1g saturates) | 15g carbs (13g total sugars) | 2g fibre

PEACH CRUMBLE

Again, you shouldn't be eating this every day. But if you're going to treat your friends and family to a Sunday pudding, I promise you they will love this.

Serves 2

2 peaches, stoned
  and diced
Juice and zest of 1 lemon
1 tbsp runny honey

For the crumble topping:

15g rolled oats
15g barley flakes
15g pecan nuts, crumbled
15g sliced almonds
½ tsp cinnamon
1 tbsp runny honey

Preheat the oven to 190°C/Fan 170°/Gas 5.

Put the diced peach into a mixing bowl along with the lemon juice and zest and honey. Mix well, then divide between two ramekins.

In another mixing bowl put the oats, barley flakes, pecan nuts, almonds, cinnamon and honey, and stir to make everything come together as a crumble topping.

Top the peaches with the oaty crumble mixture and transfer the ramekins to a large-lipped baking sheet or roasting tin lined with non-stick baking paper.

Place the tray in the oven and bake for 15 minutes, until the fruit is bubbling nicely and the top has turned golden brown.

Per serving 253 cals | 6g protein | 11g fat (1g saturates) | 31g carbs (21g total sugars) | 5g fibre

BLACK BEAN BROWNIES

Black beans? In brownies? That was my reaction when I first made them too. But, oh my!
They're so good. The beans help make them really rich and give them a nice moist texture.

Makes 9 portions

1 x 400g tin black beans, drained and rinsed
50g cocoa powder
50g rolled oats
50g brown rice flour
2 tsp baking powder
4 large eggs
4 tbsp almond milk
6 tbsp maple syrup
50g dark chocolate (90%), chopped
Pinch of salt

Preheat the oven to 180°C/Fan 160°/Gas 4.

Place the black beans, cocoa, oats, rice flour, baking powder, eggs, almond milk, maple syrup and a pinch of salt into the large bowl of a food processor. Blitz everything together for 3–4 minutes; you really want it to be as smooth as possible. Stop blitzing occasionally and scrape the mixture down the sides of the bowl to incorporate everything.

Stir through the chopped chocolate and transfer to a 20cm square cake tin lined with non-stick baking paper. Gently level the mixture out and pop it into the oven to bake for 20 minutes.

Check to see if it is done by using a cocktail stick or skewer inserted into the centre – if it comes out clean, then the cake is done. If it still has batter on it, return the cake to the oven for another 3–4 minutes before checking again.

Allow to cool for 10 minutes in the tin before using the baking paper to help lift it out. Remove the baking paper and place the cake on a wire rack to fully cool.

Once it has cooled down to room temperature, you can slice it into nine portions. These brownies are also great for the freezer, which makes it a very handy snack!

Per serving 187 cals | 8g protein | 6g fat (2g saturates) | 23g carbs (9g total sugars) | 4g fibre

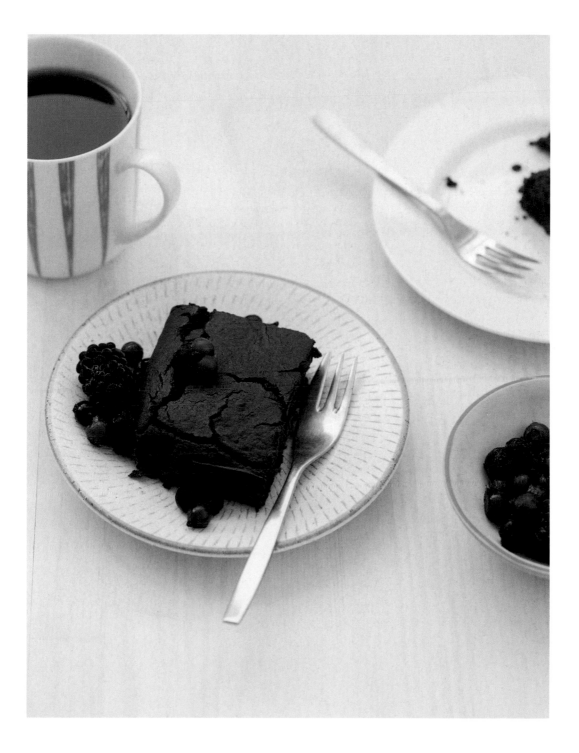

DATE BALLS

When my partner, Al, first tried these, he refused to believe they were healthy because of how delicious they are. Try them for yourself and you'll get where he's coming from.

Makes 12

100g whole blanched almonds
100g dates, pitted
2 tbsp sugar-free cocoa powder

Place the almonds and dates in a mixing bowl and boil a kettle of water. Soak them in enough boiling water to cover them and leave them for 1 hour to soften.

Drain and place the softened fruit and nuts in a food processor along with the cocoa powder. Blitz until you have a smooth-ish paste. You will need to stop and scrape the sides of the food processor down every now and again – as there isn't much moisture, the mixture will need a little help to keep moving.

Take generous teaspoons of the mix and shape it in your hands into round bites. You may find having slightly damp hands can help with the rolling.

Store the snack balls – not touching, if you can – in an airtight tub in the fridge to set their shape. A really yummy chocolatey treat!

Per serving 82 cals | 3g protein | 5g fat (1g saturates) | 6g carbs (6g total sugars) | 2g fibre

COCONUT FLAPJACK

As you can see, these are packed with great ingredients, but remember that small is beautiful and you should not be eating the entire tray! Save for emergencies when you absolutely need a little blood sugar boost.

Makes 8

150g rolled oats
50g desiccated coconut
50g coconut flakes
50g flaked almonds, roughly chopped
90g dried cherries, roughly chopped (or raisins if you can't get hold of cherries)
2 tsp ground ginger
120ml maple syrup
3 ripe bananas
2 egg whites, whisked

Preheat the oven to 170°C/Fan 150°C/Gas 3.

Place the oats, both types of coconut, almonds, cherries and ground ginger into a large mixing bowl.

Blitz the maple syrup, bananas and egg whites in a food processor to fully combine, and add to the dry ingredients. Mix everything well to make sure it's all coated.

Transfer to a 23cm cake tin lined with non-stick baking paper. Spread out the flapjack mix, pressing down gently to get it to fill the base of the tin.

Pop it into the oven to bake for 20–25 minutes. You want the edges to be lightly golden and the centre still slightly springy.

Allow to cool in the tin for 15 minutes before you lift it out. Remove the baking paper and let the flapjack fully cool on a wire rack. Cut into eight even slices.

Per serving 310 cals | 6g protein | 13g fat (7g saturates) | 40g carbs (23g total sugars) | 4g fibre

INDEX

fishcakes with steamed greens 197–8

hot and sour veggie noodle soup 223

spicy poached chicken broth 174

sweet potato quiche with salmon, dill and garden peas 182

vegetable red Thai curry 149

peppers

baked falafel salad 186

courgette and green pepper pad thai 136

deconstructed burrito bowl 231

grilled salmon and ratatouille 141

hot and sour veggie noodle soup 223

Italian-style chicken tray bake 146

peanut rice noodles 226

pork goulash 171

spicy Mexican omelette 128

spicy prawn, black bean and pepper salad 154

spicy turkey and quinoa stuffed peppers 204–5

turkey meatball tray bake 163

vegetable and lentil shepherd's pie 199

veggie fajita on cauliflower rice 185

veggie noodle stir-fry 142

periods 47, 80

personal trainers 29, 87

photos 39

pilates 93

plateauing 44, 64

pomegranate seeds

beetroot, cranberry and pomegranate salad with lime and balsamic dressing 224

fruit jelly 237

popcorn 73

pork goulash 171

porridge, buckwheat with orange and cinnamon 129

portion control 48, 50, 67–8

positivity 7, 14, 15, 24, 25–6, 40–1, 64, 79 see also affirmations

potatoes 74

prawns

fish stew 184

prawn chilli pancakes and cucumber salad 200

spicy prawn, black bean and pepper salad 154

protein 74

pulses 73 see also beans

Q

quinoa

deconstructed burrito bowl 231

nutrition 74

spicy turkey and quinoa stuffed peppers 204–5

veggie sushi with quinoa 228

R

raspberries

fruit lollies 236

raspberry sorbet 234

zesty zero cocktail 238

raspberry ketones 68

realism 41–2

red lentil and spinach dhal 179

relaxation 65

restaurants 79, 80–2

rewards 29, 47

rice 74

Riley, Lisa

her journey 8, 39–41

pantomime 87

personal journey 67, 69

skin surgery 18, 28–9

S

salads

baked falafel salad 186

beetroot, cranberry and pomegranate salad with lime and balsamic dressing 224

coconut chicken salad 178

grilled honey salmon salad with beetroot and pine nuts 176

prawn chilli pancakes and cucumber salad 200

smoked trout salad 140

spicy prawn, black bean and pepper salad 154

salmon

fishcakes with steamed greens 197–8

grilled honey salmon salad with beetroot and pine nuts 176

grilled salmon and ratatouille 141

skinny omelette wraps 220

sweet potato quiche with salmon, dill and garden peas 182

scales and weighing 45

scallops, seared scallops and sweetcorn chowder 158

seeds

beetroot, cranberry and pomegranate salad with lime and balsamic dressing 224

superfood granola with smashed banana and yoghurt 214

self-care 18–19, 28, 29, 31, 51, 65–6

self-esteem 65–6

self-judgement 14–15, 29, 40–1, 44–5

shepherd's pie, vegetable and lentil 199

shopping for food 52–3, 76

short-on-time workout 116

sleep 19

smoked trout salad 140

smoking 69

snacks 73–4, 76

sorbet, raspberry 234

soups

all green soup 132

celeriac and apple soup with chilli oatcakes 130

hot and sour veggie noodle soup 223

minestrone soup 135

miso soup with courgette and sweet potato noodles 227

mushroom ramen 138

seared scallops and sweetcorn chowder 158

white bean and garlic soup 133

spices 124

spinach

chickpea and spinach curry 156

USEFUL RESOURCES

NHS CHOICES LIVE WELL – www.nhs.uk/livewell – has information on healthy eating, weight-loss plans and support communities, as well as a calorie checker.

WEIGHT CONCERN – www.weightconcern.org.uk – provides excellent information on obesity issues, including a section on children's health and a BMI calculator.

WEIGHT LOSS RESOURCES – www.weightlossresources.co.uk – provides excellent information on weight loss, fitness and healthy eating as well as a comprehensive calorie database and a personalized weight-loss programme.

DIABETES UK – www.diabetes.org.uk – is the leading charity for people with diabetes, providing authoritative information on living with diabetes, including sections for children, teenagers and young adults.

BEAT (BEAT EATING DISORDERS) – www.b-eat.co.uk – provides helplines, online support and a network of UK-wide self-help groups, as well as downloadable information sheets and booklets.

To find a registered nutritionist visit www.associationfornutrition.org.

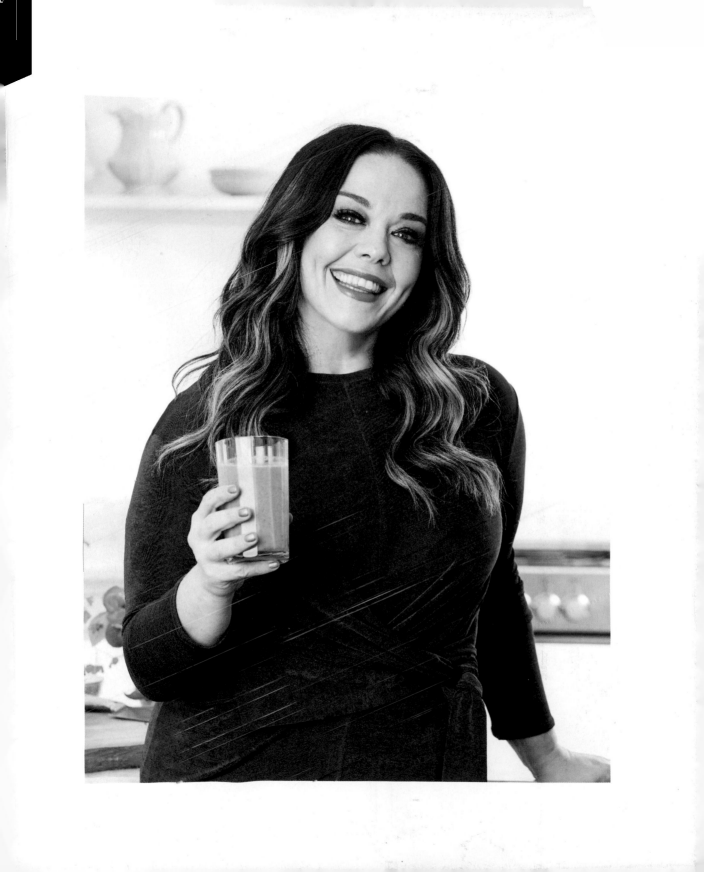

THANK YOUS

Thank you to Jordan, for continuing to help me share my ultimate passion, for showing it is possible, and for helping other people strive to be who they want to be. Thank you for letting me cry, and then cry some more. That's all thanks to you. It is allowed. And why? For the amount of times you've seen my new boobs.

Thank you to Ione. You believe in what matters, and those are always the people I adore in life. Thanks for embracing my giddiness. For that you deserve the world, and you're getting that with your new bundle of joy. #enjoy

Thank you to all the Loose Women (my loose ladies). You are like the best recipe with the best ingredients (I don't know how healthy we are though?). There's something for everyone because we're all so individual. Every mouthful of flavoursome time spent with you all means so much, and you always make me laugh and cry. #itsgoodtoshare

Thank you to Phil Dale and Courtney. Well, we've done it again. With each other's strength we get to where we want to be. We are like the best conga ever – we just keep on going. #dreamteam

Thanks to Shirley Patton at ITV, you are class in a glass. You knew how passionate I am from the second you met me, and for this I am so touched.

Thanks to my wonderful granddad for continuously fighting my corner even when you were fighting your last days on earth. Your hand went cold but your heart will be forever warm thanks to your strength and joy for life.

Thank you to Jakey and Joshua, the love I feel for you both is explosive. I love your innocence, and when you shout 'Lee-Lee, you're not fat any more' in supermarkets as loudly as you can it never fails to make me smile. #thanksforremindingmeboys

Thanks to my passport, for giving me the most unbelievable amount of happiness. It's better to be addicted to stamps than to custard creams. You've taken me to places I never knew existed except in books and movies. You opened my eyes to the REAL person I am, not the one I was hiding behind for so many years. Travelling is about finding those things you never knew you were looking for. My glass is no longer full of wine with no memory. My glass is now full of love for everything I've learned on my travels.

Thanks to everyone that has joined me on my journey, and also those who have embarked upon their own life-changing journeys. I didn't ever imagine in a million years that I would be able to create such an incredible community full of positive, happy people. I love hearing all your stories. They constantly make me feel inspired and proud, and often make me cry, but in a really, really great way. #youbloodyrock

Loads of love,
Lisa xxx